VITAL
STATISTICS:
AN INTRODUCTION TO HEALTH-SCIENCE STATISTICS

VITAL
STATISTICS:
AN INTRODUCTION TO HEALTH-SCIENCE STATISTICS

STEPHEN McKENZIE

BA(Psych)(Hons) PhD(Psych)

Research and Evaluation Officer, *Healthy Together*
preventive health initiative, City of Greater Geelong, Victoria

With contributed chapters by

DEAN McKENZIE

BA(Psych)(Hons) PhD(Psych Epidemiology)

Senior Research Fellow and NHMRC Postdoctoral Fellow,
Monash University, Melbourne, Victoria
NHMRC Postdoctoral Fellow and Honorary Fellow,
Murdoch Childrens Research Institute,
Royal Children's Hospital, Melbourne, Victoria

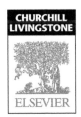

Sydney Edinburgh London New York Philadelphia St Louis Toronto

ELSEVIER

Churchill Livingstone is an imprint of Elsevier

Elsevier Australia. ACN 001 002 357
(a division of Reed International Books Australia Pty Ltd)
Tower 1, 475 Victoria Avenue, Chatswood, NSW 2067

National Library of Australia Cataloguing-in-Publication Data

Author: McKenzie, Stephen.

Title: Vital statistics : an introduction to health science statistics / Stephen McKenzie ;
Dean McKenzie.

ISBN: 9780729541497 (pbk.)

Subjects: Medical statistics. Health status indicators.

Other Authors/Contributors: McKenzie, Dean.

Dewey Number: 610.72

Publisher: Luisa Cecotti
Developmental Editors: Amanda Lucas and Neli Bryant
Project Coordinators: Geraldine Minto and Nayagi Athmanathan
Edited by Carol Natsis
Proofread by Tim Learner
Cover and internal design by studioemma
Index by Robert Swanson
Typeset by Toppan Best-set Premedia Limited, China
Printed in Australia
Transferred to digital printing 2014

Contents

Foreword

Students of health sciences are commonly required to have a basic understanding of statistics. For the more mathematically inclined, this will be easily acquired and there are many existing textbooks that will serve their needs well. However, for others learning about statistics will be an onerous task that may not seem directly relevant to their goal of becoming a health practitioner. To make statistics interesting, relevant and accessible for these students is a continuing challenge for their teachers. Having a suitable textbook that can motivate, inspire and explain complex concepts in plain language would be a big help. This new book by the McKenzie brothers does just that. It reflects many years of experience in explaining statistics to students and practitioners.

This textbook is written more in the tradition of popular science rather than in the usual textbook style. The authors have considered the needs of future health practitioners, who will be consumers rather than producers of statistics. The text is remarkably free of equations, and, when they are introduced, they are also explained in simple words.

There are lots of illustrative examples from the authors' own experiences of analysing health data, as well as some interesting historical ones. The interest level of the material is another key to its success. Anyone browsing through the text is sure to find interesting snippets that will lead them to want to read more. The humorous tone of the text also stands out as a distinguishing feature and adds to the motivation to keep reading.

I hope and expect that this new textbook will infect many health science students with the authors' obvious love of the topic and lead them to want to learn more. In particular, I hope that they see the value of statistics to evidence-based professional practice and become better practitioners as a consequence.

Anthony Jorm PhD DSc
Professorial Fellow, Melbourne School of Population Health,
University of Melbourne, Victoria

Preface

The journey is the thing.
HOMER

Statistical literacy is no longer only important for professional statisticians, scientists, gamblers and statistics students. It is now becoming as important for success in our computerised society as written literacy was to society when the printing press was invented. Unfortunately statistics books tend to teach statistics as an academic discipline, rather than as a modern life skill. The basic concepts of statistics actually include such practical universals as probability, which most of us already expertly employ, whether we realise it or not. We do not usually cross a road or buy a car or get married unless we are reasonably confident of success — in other words, if our subconscious calculation of probable success exceeds our personal criterion for action. This is a statistics book that you can take home and introduce to your family and friends, as well as to your fellow health-science students and work colleagues. It is broadly and practically useful for people studying or working in a wide range of health sciences, as well as for many other people.

Vital Statistics is a friendly, familiar and foolproof, or at least fool-resistant (hardly anything is completely foolproof), introduction or re-introduction to applied statistical literacy. Each action-packed episode includes descriptions of principles relevant to both real life and real health science that underlie even the most seemingly friendless statistics. This is a relatively small and easy-to-read book that will painlessly introduce you to statistical basics, or remind you of them, before guiding you through more demanding statistical challenges. There are therefore as few full-frontal formulas as possible, and they are translated into English — or something very close to it — to help them come alive for you.

Restricting a working knowledge of the language of information to statistical specialists is similar to restricting a working knowledge of written language to medieval monks — it risks leaving all the rest of us in an information Dark Age. Here then is the statistical equivalent of the Volkswagen Beetle, the Mini-Minor, the FJ Holden and Model T Ford — a people's statistics book. The following pages will provide you with answers to questions that you may have previously asked (but not had answered) or possibly never even thought of asking, and they will take you on a step-by-step journey to a statistically significant adventure.

Stephen McKenzie
Geelong, September 2012

Acknowledgments

Stephen McKenzie would like to thank his students at Northern Territory University (now Charles Darwin University) in 1988 who inspired this book's conception by demonstrating that there was and is a vital need for it. He would also like to thank his brother Dean (first author of Chapters 7 and 10, second author of Chapter 9 and author of Chapter 14), everyone at Elsevier who helped produce this book, the manuscript reviewers and others who facilitated this book's birth by helping transform an idea into a reality.

The responsibility for all opinions and any errors rests solely with the author(s) of the requisite chapters.

Stephen McKenzie
Geelong, September 2012

Dean McKenzie was supported by an Australian Government National Health and Medical Research Council (NHMRC) Public Health Training (Postdoctoral) Fellowship. He would like to thank his wife, Maria; his family; his colleagues at the Department of Epidemiology and Preventive Medicine at Monash University, and at the Centre for Adolescent Health, Murdoch Childrens Research Institute, Royal Children's Hospital, Melbourne; the staff of the Ian Potter Library, Alfred Hospital, and of the libraries at Monash University, University of Melbourne and Deakin University, and of the State Library of Victoria. He would like to thank his brother Stephen for inviting him to be a contributor, everyone at Elsevier who helped to produce this book, the manuscript reviewers and all of his teachers and students.

Dean McKenzie
Melbourne, September 2012

Reviewers

Anthony Bedford BAppSci(Mathematics Hons) PhD
Associate Professor, Deputy Head, Learning and Teaching, School of Mathematical and Geospatial Sciences, RMIT University, Melbourne, Victoria

Simon Boag PhD
Senior Lecturer, Department of Psychology, Macquarie University, Sydney, New South Wales

CB Del Mar MA MB BChir MD FRACGP FAFPHM
Professor of Public Health, Faculty of Health Sciences and Medicine, Bond University, Gold Coast, Queensland

Daniel Exeter BA MA(Hons) PhD
Senior Lecturer, The University of Auckland, New Zealand

Phil Hider FAFPHM(RACP) FNZCPHM
Public Health Physician, Canterbury District Health Board and University of Otago, Christchurch, New Zealand

Johnson Mak PhD FASM
ARC Future Fellow, Chair in Infectious Diseases, Professor School of Medicine, Deakin University, Melbourne, Victoria
Head, HIV and Emerging Viruses Laboratory, CSIRO Australian Animal Health Laboratory (AAHL), Geelong, Victoria

Elizabeth Manias RN MPharm MNursStud PhD FRCNA MPSA MSHPA
Professor, Melbourne School of Health Sciences, The University of Melbourne, Victoria

Judy Mullan PhD
Senior Lecturer, Graduate School of Medicine, University of Wollongong, New South Wales

Shawn Somerset PhD RPHN
Associate Professor of Public Health, School of Allied and Public Health, Australian Catholic University, Brisbane, Queensland

David Stanley NursD MSc(HS) BA(Ng) DipHE(Nursing) RN RM
Associate Professor, School of Population Health, University of Western Australia, Perth

Kerrianne Watt BSc(Hons Psych) PhD
Associate Professor, Discipline of Public Health and Tropical Medicine, School of Public Health, Tropical Medicine and Rehabilitation Sciences, James Cook University, Townsville, Queensland

To our parents, Diana and Graham,
who inspired and began our conceptions,
births and creations

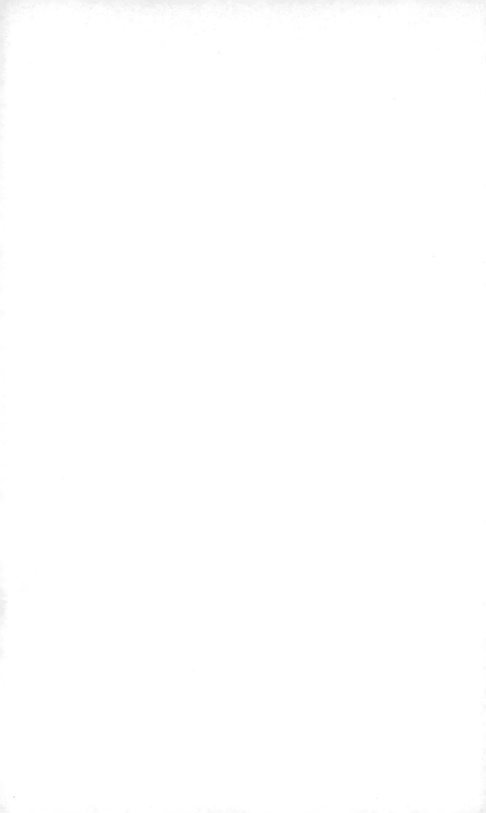

CHAPTER 1

A FOOL-RESISTANT INTRODUCTION TO STATISTICS

(Hardly anything is foolproof.)

OBJECTIVES

After carefully reading this chapter, you will:

- recognise that statistical literacy is becoming as important in our increasingly complex age as written literacy

- understand the basic purpose and nature of statistics

- realise that statistics have interesting uses in the real world, as well as perhaps not quite as interesting uses in classrooms and laboratories

- know how to emulate some interesting real-world uses of statistics that deserve to be emulated

- know how to avoid some interesting real-world misuses of statistics that deserve to be avoided

- understand that statistics are, or can be, our friend.

Introduction

A lot of otherwise mostly happy people are mostly unhappy about statistics. Unfortunately many of these people are working at jobs or enrolled in courses or living lives that involve constant exposure to statistics. This means that there are many millions of people living in statistical discomfort, misery or denial. There was a time when it was perfectly possible to live a long and fruitful life without any knowledge whatsoever of statistics. Indeed, even now it is rumoured that there are people in the remoter areas of our planet who have enjoyed a basically unchanged lifestyle for more than 40,000 years. Perhaps these fortunate few can still sleep peacefully at night with only the fuzziest notions of normal distributions or arithmetic means, but such people are modern-world outliers — exceptions to the modern norm.

There is nothing necessarily wrong with being an outlier. Indeed, if not for the outliers who realised the life-changing potential of fire and the wheel and the computer, we would still be in caves, for better or for worse. Whether or not our foray into technology was a good move is not the point. What is becoming increasingly vital to us all now is the realisation that the flow of information in our increasingly technological age is rapidly getting so complicated that there is a real risk that an underclass of information illiterates is being created. Those of us who missed out on fully learning the language of information at our schools, universities or jobs are now in danger of being distanced from the shared public domain reality that underlies much of our shared lives, in the same way that ordinary illiterates were distanced from information-sharing opportunities when the printing press was invented circa 1440.

It has been calculated that a person reading the weekend edition of a major metropolitan newspaper is exposed over that weekend to as much information as a person living several centuries ago was exposed to in their entire lifetime. The recent proliferation of statistics courses and statistical components in non-statistics courses reflects this ever-increasing practical need to keep up with the Information Age Joneses. *Vital Statistics* will provide you with enough general and health-science-specific statistical knowledge and confidence to safely and happily go as far as you would like to go on the new information superhighway.

What statistics really are and how they can help

The ever-increasing complexity of the technical demands of life on our modern planet is reflected in the rapidly expanding number of courses that now require some knowledge of statistics. Courses in a wide range of health sciences now routinely require what can seem to at least some intending health professionals to be a formidable understanding of sometimes strange and scary concepts.

When teaching inferential statistics to first-year health profession students at Darwin's then newly evolved Northern Territory University, it became obvious that it is not easy to persuade health-science students, professionals or indeed anybody else that to be a good health professional they need a steady grasp of concepts such as the random sampling distribution of means. It was easier, however, to convince health-science students, and others, that the probability theory that underlies the random sampling distribution of means is actually relevant to virtually everybody. This is true, whether you are a current or impending general practitioner, specialist, nurse, psychologist, health system administrator or even a professional or amateur gambler — a player of life's odds. What is the likely evidence-based outcome if my patients get a particular drug, operation, therapy or case-mix funding system? What is the likely evidence-based outcome if I get married to a particular person, or place all of my meagre house-deposit funds on a particular roulette wheel number?

Statistics: what's in them for me?

There are genuine reasons why a working knowledge of statistical concepts will greatly and practically benefit you as a current or impending health-science professional, and these reasons are even more important than you may currently realise. A working knowledge of statistical principles will benefit you far more broadly than just helping you do well in a course that officially or unofficially expects you to understand statistics. Understanding at least the basic principles underlying statistics is a vital modern life skill that will help you to genuinely understand the information that we are all exposed to every day, as well as to understand your professionally relevant information.

In 1954 Darrel Huff wrote what is probably the world's only statistics book bestseller to date, and it is still in print — the descriptive statistics classic *How to Lie with Statistics*.[1] The aim of this book was not to help people to use information to lie, but rather how to recognise and therefore be protected from statistical lies. Disinformation can be an insidious problem for us if we do not know what form it takes, and it could even be said that there is an epidemic of disinformation infecting our modern world. In 1954 descriptive statistical literacy was all that you needed for a competitive edge in coping with the information demands of the day. The world and its information complexity have changed, so that now we also often need to understand inferential statistics, whether we know what they are called or not, so keep reading!

The purpose of statistics

Being continually exposed to statistics when you do not understand or like them is like being in any other kind of bad relationship. The simplest solution to this common predicament is to change our attitude rather than change what we are in a bad relationship with. If the idea of statistics fills you with terror or sarcasm, do not worry; they have a similar effect on most people and this is probably not the result of some deep flaw in your character or karma. Most of us were inadvertently taught our bad statistical attitude at school, where we (well, many of us) learned to fear mathematical symbols even more than we feared sarcasm or beatings. This relates to the perfectly sensible survival law that things that are not what they seem tend to be dangerous. This principle applies to the tips of icebergs, Trojan horses and sarcasm, as well as to statistics.

At one level, both mathematics and statistics *seem* to be about what they are not. At first glance, statistical symbols such as epsilons and alphas might seem Greek to you, especially if you hail from Athens, but they actually have a saving grace, which probably nobody told you about at school, and that is that, deep down, statistics actually *mean something*.

Statistics exist to help people, including you, understand information. Information is inherently interesting as well as important even to non-statisticians, and it offers you powerful survival, entertainment and educational possibilities. The sound of a nearby twig snapping as you drink from a stream gives you only enough information to want to know more. The sight of a sabre-toothed tiger rushing at you, however, gives you enough relevant information to justify acting. The sight of a wombat or snail approaching you gives you enough relevant information to justify not acting.

Statistics as evidence

Statistics provides a tool kit that can help us describe and understand information. As such, it can conveniently be divided into two types: descriptive statistics, which consists of aids to the presentation and digestion of raw information; and inferential statistics, which uses probability theory to extrapolate information from samples to populations — from a few cases of something to all cases of it. A sample is like a taste of a wine before you buy a whole bottle of it. A population is like the bottle.

We all engage in informal inferential statistics continuously, even if we do not have a formal knowledge of it, and fortunately this is usually a painless and often useful procedure. When we make a generalisation about a life experience, we are informally, and often inaccurately, using inferential statistics. If we go to a restaurant twice and like it both times, we often come up with an extrapolation of our sample data along the lines of 'This is a good restaurant!'. Maybe it is and maybe it is not, and if we keep going back to the restaurant, and therefore increasing our sample size, then our inference — our generalisation — will become increasingly more accurate. Formal health-science decision making uses a similar common-sense evidence-based principle, and this has been described in an article on the history of medical decisions as originating in:

1. a recognition of the need for data as demonstrable evidence
2. the development of probability theory (mainly based on games of chance)
3. the development of formal inference procedures.[2]

There are many examples of the evidence-based process at work in the health sciences, and some relevant and interesting examples of these in particular statistical contexts are provided in the following chapters. An interesting evidence-based health-science statistical aperitif to sustain you until the main course is an Australian article that reports research, based on data from 175 countries, on the relationship between economic prosperity (as measured by gross domestic product, GDP), optimal body weight (as measured by a body mass index, BMI) and other factors. It is perhaps commonly assumed that as economic prosperity increases so does body weight, but the evidence-based information picture is actually more complex, more interesting and potentially more useful to a wide range of health sciences. Most countries do not have an average BMI in the optimal healthy weight range, and, of a subgroup of economically prosperous countries, those with more equally distributed prosperity (due to increased market regulation) had fewer people above the optimal weight range.[3]

Some useful statistical tips

Before consummating your relationship with statistics, it will be useful for you to know just what 'statistics' (singular) actually is, as well as what 'statistics' (plural) are. Singular 'statistics' refers to the science of summarising — describing, drawing conclusions and generalising from data — in a rigorous and orderly fashion. Plural 'statistics' refers to particular statistical tools that have been developed by the science of statistics and are used in its application.

A 'datum' is a single observation or measurement: for example, age, sex, hair colour, length of nose, type of medication being taken, football team barracked for, or level of a particular neurotransmitter substance in the brain. A datum, like a wolf, tends to hang out in packs with others of its kind, and these are known collectively as 'data'. Information is of no real use to anyone unless there is some effective means of disseminating it. To adapt a famous observation by Marshall McLuhan, statistics is the medium and also the message.[4]

Even though statistics might at least occasionally seem like an infinite series of meaningless or even obnoxious arbitrary events, they are also much more. Statistics, like mathematics and love, contain layers of meaning. Statistical tools allow us to understand information by helping us to summarise and see patterns within it, such as patterns of associations or patterns of differences. Statistics can therefore be our passport to the science and also the art of information management. To gain a working knowledge of the art of statistical science, and the science of statistical art, please read on.

Statistics in the health sciences: background

Statistics can be enormously helpful to us, whatever our field, and the practical requirements of our field can be a great motivator for us to understand and apply the statistics that are particularly relevant to it. There have been some very special cases of people who have developed or helped to develop statistical methodologies that accelerated the growth of knowledge in their special area of interest. A wheat farmer in the Australian or Canadian or Ukrainian wheat belt might not feel an overwhelming need to understand the principles of statistical analysis, especially in a good year, but such principles are far more relevant and potentially profitable to such farmers than they might realise. It can be useful to remember that statistical tools were devised by real (and often interesting) people, to meet real (and often interesting) needs (Box 1.1).

Box 1.1 Some real and interesting statistical needs and the people who met them

The great English statistician Sir Ronald Fisher (1890–1962) (Fig 1.1) developed a key statistical technique, called the analysis of variance (ANOVA), directly in response to the strong, if then unrealised, need of wheat farmers for a suitably fertile statistic. ANOVA is a technique that reveals whether apparent differences between group average scores, such as annual wheat yields, are indeed real, and its development directly led to the improvement of world wheat harvests. This great statistical discovery objectively showed whether apparent improvements in wheat yields, based on a series of modifications to wheat-growing practices, were statistically meaningful, and therefore worth introducing into wheat-farming standard practice. ANOVA is described more fully in Chapter 8.

Florence Nightingale (Fig 1.2), whose name might be more familiar to you than that of Sir Ronald Fisher, was also inspired by the largely unrealised demands for her profession in the nineteenth century to apply and develop an appropriate and powerfully practical statistical methodology. Florence Nightingale is, of course, a famous health professional, who became known for helping injured soldiers and others during the Crimean War. Her enormous contribution to humanity in that situation and others was not just the result of her great compassion and energy; it was also due to her recognition that such qualities can be far more useful when applied in conjunction with a statistical scientist's ability to see and meet a need.

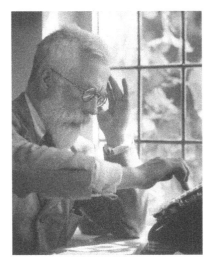

Fig 1.1 **Sir Ronald Fisher, a great statistical pioneer** (Courtesy RA Fisher Memorial Trust)

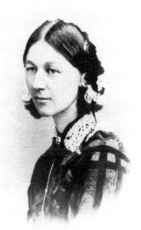

Fig 1.2 **Florence Nightingale, a great statistical pioneer** (From Boyd J. Florence Nightingale and Elizabeth Blackwell. *The Lancet*. 2009;373(9674), Fig 2.)

Statistics in the health sciences: foreground

If you are involved in the health sciences, and you have bought or borrowed this book, you are in a wonderful position to apply statistical principles and tools to a highly valuable area, and applying statistics to something valuable and personally relevant will help them to come alive. Statistical literacy will help you in any field of the health sciences, and it will help you whether your area is predominately clinical, research-related or administrative, because research informs practice and practice informs research. Statistical literacy will help you to understand as well as to conduct relevant research and evidence-based clinical practice; it will be of great help in your professional life as well as enabling you to pass statistics exams. The use of evidence-based medicine, for example, can lead you to run fewer unnecessary tests, whether you are a doctor, a nurse, a psychologist or anyone else with a practical or theoretical interest in health science.

Some interesting health-science uses and abuses of statistics

Statistics can be of great benefit to us, whether as health professionals, wheat farmers or any other active members of the modern human race. Some broad examples of statistics in action that are particularly relevant to health professionals are given in this section. These examples illustrate the great potential power and fascinating applicability of statistics to the real world, and to the real health-science world. They also illustrate the sometimes intriguing damage that these statistics can cause if they are used unwisely. These examples are also intended to give you some preliminary familiarity with important basic statistical principles (to be described in more detail in later chapters) in contexts that relate research to clinical and other real-life applications.

An early example

An interesting early attempt at using the objectivity of statistics to provide potentially life-changing health information to health consumers involved a trial comparing the results of a vegetable and water diet with a 'Royal' diet of meat and wine. This study was reported in the Bible (Daniel 1:12–16). Daniel suggests to the guards that he and his three companions be given nothing but vegetables to eat and water to drink so as to compare the effects of this diet with a far more regal one. At the end of a 10-day 'study period', the four experimental participants looked in much better health than the young men who had been given the regal diet. Daniel's choice of methodological paradigm was governed, as such choices often still are, by practical considerations: in this case, the young men who had been eating regal rations might not have been all that interested in giving them up, especially without convincing empirical evidence that there is a healthier way to eat. Daniel could also have explored his research and clinical interest by looking at associations, rather than at differences, between groups: for example, by calculating the relationship between the effect on health of regal rations and other health-associated factors, such as age and stress levels. Undoubtedly, however, Daniel was aware of the important statistical principle that, just because a factor is associated with health, this does not mean that it has influenced health, and thus he wisely chose an experimental methodology.

A modern example

A more recent study that is distantly related to the above biblical one was reported by the CSIRO in Adelaide, Australia, in 2009.[5] This study combined the interests of several health sciences by comparing the mood and cognitive effects, as well as the weight-loss effects, of a low-carb, high-fat Atkins-style diet with a high-carb, low-fat diet. Participants in this study were tested initially, then assigned one of these two diets and then tested again after 12 months. The results of the study revealed that both weight loss and cognition level did not differ meaningfully between the two groups of dieters, but mood (depression, anxiety) was significantly worse for the low-carb, high-fat group. This means that a low-carb, high-fat Atkins-style diet is neither better nor worse at facilitating weight loss than is a high-carb, low-fat diet, and also that the Atkins-style diet negatively effects mood.

These findings give us even more food for thought than simply the very pertinent information that we can use to inform our dieting choices. Findings such as this demonstrate the considerable discrepancy that can exist between what people think is true and what objective statistical evidence shows is true.

There is a contemporary, widespread common perception that low-carb diets are particularly effective for facilitating weight loss. Contemporary, widespread common perceptions are not necessarily factually based, because they are not necessarily based on a reasoned statistical interpretation of reasonable data. These common perceptions are often misperceptions and could reasonably be termed 'belief fashions', which can be as cyclical and as unreliable as fashions of dress or behaviour. There was a time when it was fashionable to believe that the earth was flat, and that high-carb intake is critical to elite sporting performance. Worlds and carbs generally do not change their fundamental properties quickly, but fashions and opinions generally do. The important point of the dietary experimental example is that a statistically literate person can choose not to believe in information myths and can look objectively and reasonably at the actual objective evidence.

Health-science information versus health-science disinformation

Everybody knows that antidepressants are useful for treating people with depression. Is everybody right? The new generation of antidepressants famously started out with Prozac in 1988 and are collectively known as selective serotonin reuptake inhibitors (SSRIs). They indirectly increase brain levels of neurotransmitters such as serotonin that are associated with positive mood states (which incidentally are also indirectly increased by chocolate and by love). SSRIs increase happiness-associated brain chemistry by reducing the loss (reuptake) of serotonin. Antidepressants are very commonly prescribed and are widely accepted clinically as well as popularly as being an effective and important treatment option for people with depression. Is this the whole statistical story?

A large statistical analysis performed in the UK in 2008[6] has created considerable interest in whether the efficacy of antidepressants for treating depression is a scientific truth, or a truism — a partial or convenient truth. This study combined samples that were used in many investigations of the effectiveness of antidepressants, including unpublished ones, to form a very large and unusually representative sample of antidepressant users. This method allowed conclusions about the efficacy of antidepressants to be inferred from this larger-than-usual sample and applied to the population of all antidepressant users everywhere. The results of this analysis showed that overall, despite a widespread clinical and public belief in their efficacy, antidepressants do not reduce symptoms of depression more effectively than do placebos for mild-to-moderate depression, according to a widely accepted clinical criterion.

This example illustrates the importance of separating the information wheat from the disinformation chaff. The perceptions of expert scientists and clinicians in the health sciences are not necessarily always based on a fully informed, objective appraisal of the relevant evidence. Instead these perceptions can sometimes be based mainly on the sheer weight of numbers and the scientific credibility of the people who believe in them.

Conclusion

Statistics can help us to understand what it is useful for us to understand, whether we realise it or not. Statistics are highly practical because they can help us to objectively describe, structure and understand the information that we are exposed to every day, and they can help us to objectively test our hypotheses about this information. Statistics can be especially useful to health professionals and students of health professions, because health professionals work in areas where it is vital to use information optimally — to ask and answer vital questions. The following chapters will reveal how statistics can be used optimally in a wide range of meaningful real health-science life situations.

Quick reference summary

- Statistics exist to help us understand information.
- Statistics are highly useful in our information age, and can be particularly useful for health-science students and workers.
- Understanding statistical principles is an important modern life skill.
- Singular 'statistics' refers to the science of summarising data.
- Plural 'statistics' refers to the tools developed by the science of statistics and used in its application.
- 'Data' are collections of observations or measurements, such as age, sex, hair colour, length of nose or type of medication being taken.
- Statistics are, or can be, our friend.

References

1. Huff D. *How to Lie with Statistics*. Illustrations I Geis. New York: Norton; 1954.

2. Mazur DJ. A history of evidence in medical decisions: from the diagnostic sign to Bayesian inference. *Medical Decision Making*. 2012;32(2):227-231. Epub 2012 Jan 27.

3. Egger G, Swinburn B, Islam FM. Economic growth and obesity: an interesting relationship with world-wide implications. *Economic Human Biology*. 2012;10(2):147-153. Epub 2012 Jan 20.

4. McLuhan M. *Understanding Media: the Extensions of Man*. New York: Mentor; 1964.

5. Brinkworth GD, Buckley JD, Noakes M, et al. Long-term effects of a very low-carbohydrate diet and a low-fat diet on mood and cognitive function. *Archives of Internal Medicine*. 2009;169(20):1873-1880.

6. Kirsch I, Deacon BJ, Huedo-Medina TB, et al. Initial severity and antidepressant benefits: a meta-analysis of data submitted to the food and drug administration. *PLOS Medicine*. 2008;5:260-268.

CHAPTER 2

STATISTICS AS INFORMATION

Information is the resolution of uncertainty.
CLAUDE SHANNON (1916–2001)

OBJECTIVES

After carefully reading this chapter you will:

- understand what data is and how it can be usefully represented

- know how data relates to information, and how information relates to knowledge

- understand what disinformation is and how it can be avoided

- know what the standardisation of scores means, and how this can help transform data into information

- achieve statistical wisdom.

Introduction

Statistics is an information science and it begins with the basic building blocks of data as information units. No matter how complex a statistical question is, in order to answer it successfully we firstly need to understand the basic nature of the data, and how to optimally structure it. In this modern age it is becoming increasingly likely that we will suffer from information indigestion or even disinformation overdose, unless we have a rudimentary knowledge of what information really is and how it can be gainfully employed. Statistics is a highly useful modern tool because it can provide us with enough general understanding and specific techniques to separate the information signals of the world from its disinformation noise. This chapter will introduce you to data as information building blocks and to techniques for structuring data, so that data can readily be transformed into information and then into knowledge.

Statistics is a language that can give meaning to the potential chaos of the masses of raw information that surround us and convert it into something that can be extremely useful to us and that can guide our decision-making processes, including our health-science–related decision-making processes. Descriptive statistics allows us to describe and compare phenomena that are meaningful to us, such as the incidence rates of a particular disease. Inferential statistics allows us to describe and compare relationships between phenomena, by inferring population information on the basis of information obtained from samples of these populations, such as by trialling the efficacy of a new treatment on a sample of a clinical population. Either information can occur naturally, such as the incidence rate of a particular disease, or information can be deliberately obtained by controlling and varying experimental conditions, such as by giving some people a new treatment and giving others a placebo, and then comparing their results on a suitable measure.

Data

We are exposed to information every day of our lives, and formalising this everyday concept in statistical terms allows us to describe the phenomena of life in a precise and ultimately measurable manner.

Data scales

Data can be measured on different scales, to different levels of precision. There is no one true and optimal data type, just as there is no one true and optimal knowledge type; there are just levels of data types, which vary in terms of how much information they preserve. The preservation of information is generally a good and noble aim, and when our information conditions allow it we should aspire to this ideal. Sometimes we can use a data scale that allows us to retain all of our information. Sometimes, however, we do not have the resources to maintain all that is precious to us, so we need to reduce the full range of information that our data offers. In 1946, a psychologist named Stanley Smith Stevens published definitions of four types of measurement scale (nominal, ordinal, interval and ratio), which are still widely used, and each of them offers advantages and disadvantages to the statistically literate information consumer.[1] We will discuss each of these in turn.

The nominal scale

The nominal scale is a categorical data scale in that it divides data into categories. This scale contains only rudimentary information about our phenomena of interest. The nominal scale presents information in the form of classifications into at least two categories, where there is not necessarily any meaningful relationship between the categories. An example of a nominal scale is one that represents two colours — red and purple. In this case we have two categories of information consisting of (1) red and (2) purple. It is not stated or even implied whether red is greater than purple, or better, or faster, or happier — it is just different. This could be a useful information scale if our statistical interest does not include shades of grey, or indeed shades of red or purple. A health-science example of a nominal scale is one that represents blood groups, where the categories A, B, AB and O are just different, without one being better or worse than the others.

The nominal data scale is relatively easy to conceptualise, put into operation and analyse, but using it can result in losing information, or at least mislaying it. Using a two-category nominal scale can, for example, result in the reduction of five units of levels of smoking recorded to a single unit of information, characterised as *non-smoker*. A commonly used example of data measured on a nominal scale is gender, which generally has two categories — male and female — with no relationship (statistically at least) between them, in that one is not greater than or lesser than the other. Other commonly used nominal data scales include nationality, religion, blood and colour of eyes, hair or jelly beans, none of which has a meaningful relationship between their categories. We can arbitrarily assign the number 1 to males and 2 to females, but we could just as correctly assign the number 1 to females and 2 to males. These numbers are just arbitrary codes to signify unrelated categories.

The ordinal scale

The ordinal scale can also be a categorical scale. It preserves more information about the phenomena of interest than does the nominal scale, because it includes information on relationships between categories. Runners finishing first, second and third in a race provide an example of data measured on an ordinal scale. In this case we may not have preserved all of the information available to us, such as finishing time, but we may have preserved enough information to satisfy us if our interest is merely in the comparative fastness of runners.

A commonly used example of the use of an ordinal scale is in the measurement of age. In this case typically a possible 100+ units of age information can be reduced to as few as two categories: (1) young and (2) old. How much useful information we trade for computational ease when we use this sort of scale depends on the nature of our research question. As with finishing order, with age there is a meaningful relationship between the ordinal categories of young and old, in that they can be said to be greater or lesser than each other. Phenomena measured on an ordinal scale are not necessarily equidistant, however; in other words, the difference between whatever is first in the category order and whatever is second does not have to be the same as the difference between whatever is second and whatever is third (see Box 2.1 for an example).

A health-science example of the potential non-equivalence of distances between data points measured in an ordinal scale is the commonly administered self-reported pain levels — on a scale of 1–10 — that are used by many health-science professionals. There might be a far greater distance in actual pain experienced between a reported pain level of 5 and one of 4 than there is between a reported pain level of 4 and one of 6. Even though the distance between points on an ordinal scale may not be equidistant, the relationship between these points still has meaning. A self-reported pain score of 10 is higher than a score of 5, regardless of the comparative distances between scores.

Box 2.1 **A nose is a nose is a nose**

A very general example of the potential non-equivalence of distances between data points measured on an ordinal scale relates to nose counting, and involves a famous Australian race horse's 2012 visit to Royal Ascot in the UK. Black Caviar had won all of her previous 21 races and most of them by considerable margins, but her trainer observed before a particularly important race — the Diamond Jubilee Stakes — that he did not care how much his horse won by, as long as she won. He was right, statistically speaking; the prize was the same whether his horse won by her usual wide margins or by a considerably smaller one. Black Caviar won the 2012 Diamond Jubilee Stakes by … a nose.

The interval scale

The interval scale allows us to structure information into two or more categories and to express it in terms of actual values. The intelligence test is a commonly used health-science example of an interval scale. If an intelligence test respondent obtains an overall score of 122 on a Wechsler Adult Intelligence Test Scale, this data gives us some fairly specific information about how this respondent is performing compared, for example, with one who scored 66 and with one who scored 166, but this is not the end of the statistical information story. It is not appropriate for a health professional, or for anyone else, to state that someone who scored 132 on an intelligence test is twice as intelligent as somebody who scored 66. This is because interval scales do not have true zeroes. A score of zero on an intelligence test does not, thankfully, signify zero intelligence.

Similarly, it is not possible to state that a temperature of 22°C is twice as hot as a temperature of 11°C, because the zeroes used in such scales are not true zeroes. A temperature of 0°C is 32°F, and is a very long way from absolute zero. However, the points on intelligence and temperature interval scales are equidistant. The difference between a temperature of 26°C and 18°C is exactly the same as the difference between a temperature of 18°C and 10°C. The Celsius scale, incidentally, is defined as the temperature on the Kelvin scale minus 272.15.[2]

The ratio scale

The ratio scale structures information into actual values, where proportional relationships such as 'twice as much' as and 'half as much' as can be expressed, as well as relationships such as 'greater than' or 'less than', because this scale uses a true zero. If our health-science–related research interest should happen to be in the length of javelin throws, possibly because our very expensive health-science corporate box Olympic seats are located perilously close to the javelin throwers, then the ratio scale is particularly suited to this data, because length of a javelin throw has a true zero. A javelin thrown zero metres may be considered by some statisticians, sports scientists and philosophers to be a non-throw, but thankfully we do not need to consider such a controversy here. A javelin throw of zero metres is exactly 50 metres less than a throw of 50 metres, and a throw of 25 metres is exactly half as long as a throw of 50 metres.

An example of a ratio scale that is more directly relevant to health science is blood pressure, which has a true zero. The Kelvin scale is also a ratio scale because it has an absolute zero, with zero meaning no temperature at all. Temperatures measured on the Kelvin scale can therefore be expressed as proportions such as 'twice as hot' or 'half as hot'.

The scales of data justice

An important thing to remember about types of data is that scales of measurement should be appropriate to our research and/or clinical interest. We can quantify the efficacy of a new drug treatment on a scale with the categories 'good' and 'not good', but it will probably be far more useful to obtain more information about the efficacy of the drug treatment, including information about the relationship between the data described on our scale. We could therefore define measures that more specifically quantify our interest in the efficacy of the drug treatment by constructing a scale that allows ordinal ratings of drug efficacy, or that provides a quantitative measure such as blood pressure. Being able to recognise and implement appropriate data scales is an important first step on the road to statistical literacy, and the nature of the research and/or clinical question will determine which scale best suits the presentation of our information.

Data distributions

The binomial distribution

We can begin our description of data distributions with the binomial distribution (Box 2.2), which plots the frequency of a series of binary events such as yes/no, black or white, or even yin or yang. It is possible to see many natural and human phenomena in binary terms, rather than in continuous terms, for instance in terms of black and white rather than as shades of grey. In medicine, for example, patients can be accurately diagnosed as being either pregnant or not pregnant, or even alive or dead, and these classifications work well as binary possibilities. Conceptualising patients as either sick or well can be problematically simplistic, however, compared with classifying them on a continuous scale such as that provided by the General Health Questionnaire.[3] This measure provides a broad indication of human health that is similar to what a car-roadworthiness test provides for car health.

In cases where the data is definitively binary, and not just treated as such by reducing it to two possibilities for reasons of convenience, convention or lack of imagination, the binomial distribution can be useful. If the data are innately binary (heads, tails; male, female) or are treated as such (sick, well; intelligent, not intelligent) and the size of our sample or population is fixed and known, then statistical analysis of counts and proportions will often make use of the binomial distribution.

The normal distribution

A possibly interesting characteristic of nature, and of human nature, is that measurements of its constituent phenomena often form normal distributions. A possibly interesting characteristic of normal distributions is that normally distributed data contain many scores clustered around the average score, with successively fewer scores occurring at the high and low ends of the distribution. When plotted on a graph a normal distribution

Box 2.2 **A short history of the binomial distribution**

The binomial distribution was originally defined in the seventeenth century by the Swiss philosopher and mathematician Jakob (or Jacques) Bernoulli (1655–1705).[4] The Bernoulli distribution is a special case of the binomial distribution and is based on one trial — the probability of a single toss of the coin coming up heads. The binomial distribution refers to multiple trails/tosses. Examples of this type of distribution include the number of heads coming up in a series of two-up coin tosses in an Australian casino, the number of females born in a particular year out of the total population or the prevalence of a psychiatric disorder in a sample. The binomial probability formula was not published until 1712 — as *Ars Conjectandi* (The Art of Conjecturing) — eight years after Bernoulli's death.

In 1710, however, the great early statistician Dr John Arbuthnot (1667–1725) decided that it was God's plan that there be more males born than females, as men tended to have more accidents and deaths, such as in seeking food for their families.[5] Arbuthnot examined the available London birth records covering a period of 82 years and found that there were indeed more males born in each year of that period, although this does not necessarily indicate support for the 'Divine Providence' hypothesis. Interested readers are directed to Everitt.[6]

of scores resembles a two-dimensional bell in shape — high in the middle and symmetrically tapering down towards infinitely low or high scores on both sides.

Out of the myriad potential examples of phenomena that are normally distributed, one example is students' statistics examination scores, where there are a few very high and low scores and a great many middling scores. Another ubiquitous example of a normal distribution is intelligence test results, where most of us are of approximately average intelligence, at least according to intelligence tests, and few of us achieve either very high or very low scores. The weights of pills and the numbers of leaves on trees also form normal distributions.

When there are very few extreme scores in a distribution, these are often known as outliers, which simply means that these scores are much higher or lower than most of the scores in their distribution and may have come from a different distribution, possibly as the result of operator or subject error (for example, when the leads fell off in an EEG test).

It is important that we get to know our data properly before we conduct intimate statistical analyses on it, and part of this acquaintance-building process involves inspecting the nature of its distribution and checking for outliers. Outliers in our data distribution can distort the results of statistical tests, even statistical tests as simple as calculating the mean, so we need to determine whether the existence of outliers means that we need to statistically respond to them, even if only by calculating the less extreme sensitive median rather than mean. We should remember, however, that outliers may still be legitimate data points.

Normal distribution spotting

We can spot a normal distribution by observing the following character-istics in our data:

- Normal distributions are symmetrical and bell-shaped

- Normal distributions are *dense* in the centre and taper symmetrically towards their two ends.

It should be borne in mind, however, that a completely normal distribution is extremely rare and could therefore be viewed as an ideal.

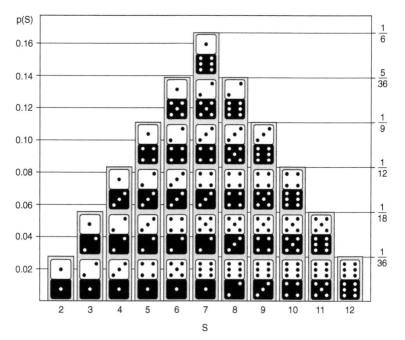

Fig 2.1   **A normal distribution of possible two-dice roll results**

Many statistical tests assume that data are normally distributed, and therefore we should be aware of whether our data are approximately normally distributed in our statistical decision making. If our data are not approximately normally distributed, this may be because the distribution is bimodal, with two humps (and roughly equivalent to the Bactrian camel) instead of the usual one hump (roughly equivalent to the dromedary). An example of a bimodal distribution is heights, where there is typically a modal hump for males and another modal hump for females.

Another cause of non-normality of our data is skewness, which can be positive or negative. This is generally not as painful as it may sound and is characterised by a positive skew pointing to a trailing off to very few high scores, or a negative skew pointing to a trailing off to very few low scores (Fig 2.3).

Some common examples of skewed data in the health sciences include: mean arterial blood pressure levels where people with various conditions have higher than average blood pressures; white blood cell count in healthy adults; and length of hospital stay where there are more shorter than longer stays.

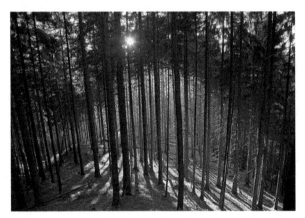

Fig 2.2   **A natural normal distribution — of woods, trees and leaves** (David Pinzer/ Flickr)

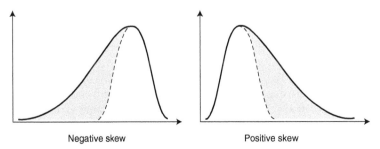

Negative skew   Positive skew

Fig 2.3   **Negative and positive skewness**

Assumption of normally distributed data

We need to know what the distribution of data looks like before we can appropriately apply statistical tests to it. This process is basically one of statistical commonsense and is functionally similar to being aware of the normal or non-normal distribution of wear on our car tyres before driving off on them. The assumption of the normal distribution of data is also important for working out the probabilities that the characteristics of our samples will be true of their underlying populations, which will be discussed in more detail in a Chapter 4.

It has been suggested that the perfectly normal distribution is a myth, but whether normal distributions are as rare as unicorns, as claimed by some theorists,[7] or as common as mules, it does not really matter, because statistical tests generally ask no more of our data than we would ask of our friends — merely that they be approximately normal. Some slight discrepancies or abnormalities or eccentricities can usually be accommodated in our statistical testing without any serious disturbance of our relationship with our data. We need to be familiar, however, with the kinds of non-normal distributions that may be lurking in our data, so that we can identify them and their level of data danger, and respond accordingly.

Variables

Statistics can be seen as the science, and also the art, of transforming data into information and of transforming information into knowledge. This applied 'alchemical' process could be seen to metaphorically begin with the base metal of our raw data, and end with the gold of knowledge that can affect people's lives. Data is extremely diverse and can include the beauty of a sunrise or the number of cars in a traffic jam, or even the number of human noses (nose counts) and their lengths.

We can conveniently divide data into two aspects:

1. the objects that we wish to study, and

2. the characteristics of the objects that we wish to study.

The measured characteristics of a variable constitute a data set of particular values. An example of an object is a human nose, which we may wish to include in our count (Box 2.3). A variable, therefore, is a measure that is expressed in terms of its values, or variability. A variable can be seen as a filing cabinet and its values as the files. A variable with only one potential value is not a variable at all, but a constant, and apart from such potential universalities as God, love and taxes, we live in a mainly variable world. If our variable is the level of beauty of a sunrise, then the variability of this variable might be defined on a scale of subjective beauty ratings. Variables can contain different types of information, depending on the

Box 2.3 **Nose variability measuring as an extension of nose counting**

A general example of a characteristic of an object that we might be interested in measuring is length of human noses. The characteristics of data are known as variables, because such characteristics vary. Nose length, for example, can vary between short, long and extremely long, if we wished to define its variability in terms of a categorical variable. Nose length can also vary in terms of discrete units of measurements such as centimetres, if we wished to define its variability as a ratio variable.

Incidentally the human nose continues to grow for as long as we live, which has consequences beyond data gathering (nose counting) and analysis, and may make immortality a less attractive option than it may otherwise appear.

type of scale upon which they were measured. The variable is therefore the basic unit of measurement that forms the building block for many statistical techniques.

Types of variable

There are two main types of variable that are commonly used in situations where the researcher is manipulating the conditions: the independent variable (which the researcher varies) and the dependent variable (which can be seen as resulting from what has been varied). The independent variable is what varies between conditions of our research and/or clinical interest and can also be described as a predictor variable or an explanatory variable. The dependent variable depends on the independent variable and can be seen as its measure. It can also be described as a criterion variable or outcome variable.

An example of this division of variables in health-science research or clinical action is one in which we may be interested in comparing the efficacy of different doses of a new antiepileptic drug that has been developed specifically for use on patients with comorbid symptoms, such as those of autism. We need an outcome measure of the efficacy this drug, such as number or severity of seizures, which is our dependent/criterion/outcome variable. We also need to vary drug dosage levels, which are the levels of our independent/predictor/explanatory variable. If we are using statistics that will provide a measure of association between variables rather than demonstrate a causal relationship between them, such as between drug dose level and degree of side effects, then we would generally not describe our variables in terms of the above typology.

Standardisation of data

It is common in the health sciences to find ourselves in research and clinical situations where we need to begin with a common scale of measurement before we can meaningfully statistically analyse relationships between sets of scores. An important principle of statistics, and also of business, is that sometimes, at least, we cannot directly compare apples with oranges, or pears with zucchinis, or data of one sort with data of another sort. It is therefore sometimes necessary to transform our data into a common language — a standardised score that includes oranges and apples — for example, by creating a common 'fruit' scale. The advantages of standardising scores are illustrated in the following statistical dramatisation:

'Hi Erin — I know that a lot of you nursing students were worried about your stats test today. How did you go?'

'Hi Jack. Well, we're not worried any more — about stats or anything else. We've all been reading a wonderful new stats book called *Vital Statistics*!'

'That's great news. I'll recommend it to all of my psychology student mates! How did you go on the test?'

'I scored 7.'

'Um, was that good?'

'The test was out of 100!'

'Oh, well maybe you should have read your book twice!'

'No need. Seven was one of the highest marks in the class — and the average was 2.5!'

'Hey, that must have been some test! I suppose that what your score really demonstrates is that raw scores don't actually mean anything. If I didn't know how your stats score compared with other people's scores, I wouldn't have known whether 7 was good or bad!'

'That's so true. You really seem to understand stats!'

'Well, at first I hated and feared them as much as most of my friends do, but then one day I was lucky enough to meet a simple stats guru who told me something I could understand — that there are general principles behind stats which make statistical details meaningful, if you look at them closely enough. Incidentally there's a terrific statistical movie on tomorrow night — *The Significant Other*. Would you like to see it with me?'

'Probably!'

As well as being a self-contained statistical romance and a shameless advertisement for this book, the above dialogue illustrates the dangers of being exposed to too much raw data, which can give you mental indigestion. To be fully digestible — meaningful — raw scores need to be cooked. This means transforming them into a scale where they are expressed in relation to other scores, in much the same way that to be meaningful people and many other life forms need to relate to other members of their species. This is a general principle of physics, as well as of life and statistics. Albert Einstein once rather famously came up with a general and also a special formula of relativity, that basically states that you cannot have movement without also having something to relate that movement to. To prevent a situation where there are as many meanings of scores as there are scores, we need a common language — a statistical lingua franca like Esperanto. As it happens, statistics provides us with a common language into which we can translate our individual scores (Box 2.4).

Percentiles

A simple way of transforming scores into a common scale is to convert them into percentiles. Erin's stats test score of 7 placed her at the 90th percentile of the stats test takers. This means that she scored higher than 90% of the students who took the stats test and that she therefore scored in the top 10%. If Erin had expressed her stats score as a percentile to Jack, rather than as a raw score, with just some elementary understanding of this common language Jack would have realised immediately that Erin had done really well.

There is a problem, however, with using percentiles as a common language with which to express scores: they do not preserve the original relationship between scores. If Erin had scored at the 90th percentile on

---

Box 2.4 **Standardisation and science fiction**

Contact is a science fiction movie that was made in 1997 and starred Jodie Foster and John Hurt. This movie was based on a novel by Carl Sagan and it was about some especially lonely and smart earthlings who decided to send messages way off into the unspeakable reaches of space to try to contact other intelligent life forms. They transformed their messages into mathematical symbols, because these are far more universal than are our non-mathematical languages. The same principle applies in statistics — we can transform our raw scores into a common language that everybody blessed with some basic statistical literacy can understand.

the test and her friend Amber had scored at the 89th percentile, Jack might have been almost as impressed with Amber's score as he was with Erin's, and maybe would have ended up going out with her instead. Percentiles can be misleading, however, because Amber actually scored only 5.5 on the test — much lower than Erin did in absolute terms, but her score was the next highest. We do not get a sense of this gap when we speak about the 90th versus the 89th percentile.

A standardised score that preserves the original relationship between raw scores, as well as showing you where a score lies in relation to other scores, will be even more useful than percentiles are. You will therefore undoubtedly be relieved, if not thrilled, to discover that there is a standard score that preserves the relationship between raw scores. Note, however, that standardising data does not make non-normally distributed data normal. This standard score is known, logically enough, as the standard score — or sometimes, the z-score.

The z-score

All you really need to know about the z-score is that it translates scores from one language (a specific measurement scale) into a common language (a general measurement scale). Although the z-score is not as famous as some of the world's other great statistical or mathematical transformation processes, such as those used in the World War II Enigma decoding project that eventually cracked the Nazis' secret military codes, it follows a similar principle. The z-score, however, is potentially as useful as the Babel fish in Douglas Adams's *The Hitchhiker's Guide to the Galaxy*. This amazingly useful, if imaginary, fish can apparently be placed painlessly into your ear, where it will then incredibly obligingly translate whatever is said to you, in whatever language, into your own language. We therefore encourage you to see the z-score as a statistical Babel fish that can standardise any score, no matter how scaly.

The underlying principle of the z-score relates to the normal data distribution that was introduced above. A z-score is a standard score that tells us how far the raw score (from which it was derived) is from the mean of its complete data distribution, given in terms of distance from the mean. This distance from the mean is expressed as standard deviation units, which will be described in more detail in Chapter 3. Fortunately for those of us who want to calculate z-scores, the normal distribution has some highly useful mathematical properties that allow us to calculate what percentage of raw scores fall below or above particular z-scores, which means that z-scores can easily be translated into percentiles. We know from the properties of the normal distribution, for example, that 15.8% of scores in it are lower than a z-score of −1, and that 15.8% of scores in it are higher than +1.

It is possible in our information-saturated age to perform z-tests, t-tests and even discriminant function analyses until we scream in the night, without having any real idea of what they actually mean. But if we can do at least some of these calculations by hand, and understand their basic principles, this will help us to understand their nature and their usefulness. We will therefore advance your practical statistical discovery mystery tour with a short z-score formula day trip, which will include a translation of it into English, or something closely resembling it. We will then provide you with an illustration of this statistic in action via a meaningful and possibly interesting example.

The formula for calculating a z-score is:

$$Z = \frac{X - M}{SD}$$

This can be translated into English as:

To calculate the z standard score, subtract the mean score of a set of scores from the individual score and then divide this by the standard deviation.

This can be illustrated by the following example:

Immediately after going to the movie *The Significant Other* with Erin, Jack unfortunately fell into a coma on his way home, possibly from the effects of too much statistical stimulation. A neuropsychologist tested Jack when he woke up in hospital the next morning to assess possible brain damage. One of the tests that was administered was the Rey Verbal Learning Auditory Test. When Jack was released from hospital later that day he visited Erin:

'Hey, Erin, I scored 5 on trial 1 of my Rey memory test!'

'That's fantastic, Jack, I think, but what does that score actually mean? You look fine, I might hastily add!'

'Good point, Erin! Well, using the original 1964 French Rey norms, we can calculate a standard score, or z-score, for my performance because my scores are normally distributed. We can then use this z-score to compare my test performance to that of other students about my age!'

'Wonderful! How?'

'That's easy. We simply subtract my raw score — 5 — from the group mean score, which we know from the comparative norm table is 8.9, which gives us 3.9. We then divide 3.9 by the standard deviation, which we know from the norm table is 1.9, and the answer is that my z-score equals 2!'

'That's great, Jack! What does it mean?'

'Well, Erin, if we compare that score to the z distribution table, which is a standardised normal distribution — and I just happen to have one in my pocket — we can see that, according to the 1964 norms, a z-score of negative 2 means that I scored lower than did almost 98% of the comparative normative population, which suggests that I'm probably brain-damaged!'

'Um, I'm sorry to hear that, Jack.'

'Don't worry! That just shows you the importance of using appropriate norms. According to more recent and more local norms[8] my z-score is approximately 0, which means that I'm fine!'

'That's terrific!'

This example illustrates the basic principle underlying the value of standardising scores: we need a common language that ensures that one person is not talking about apples while another is hearing oranges, because both are discussing fruit.

Conclusion

You have been introduced in this chapter to the notion that statistics are an information science, and to some of the important characteristics of the scientific and effective use of information. Chapter 3 will introduce you to one of the two major types of statistics — descriptive statistics. It will provide you with enough theoretical and practical knowledge of the detail and underlying principles of descriptive statistics to protect you from descriptive statistical ignorance and deceit (other people's and your own!).

Quick reference summary

- Statistics is an information science and it begins with the basic building blocks of data as information units.

- Data can be measured on different scales, to different levels of precision, and a common division of data is into nominal, ordinal, interval and ratio scales.

- The binomial distribution plots the frequency data of a series of binary events such as yes/no, black or white, or even yin or yang.

- Measurements of human and other forms of nature tend to form normal distributions.

- Normally distributed data contain many scores clustered around the average score, with successively fewer scores occurring at the high and low ends of the distribution.

- A variable is a measure that is expressed in terms of its values, or variability. A variable can be seen as a filing cabinet and its values as the files.

- In the health sciences we commonly need a common scale of measurement to statistically analyse relationships between sets of scores in a meaningful way.

- Common ways of standardising scores include the calculation of percentiles and z-scores.

References

1. Stevens SS. On the theory of scales and measurement. *Science.* 1946;102:667-680.

2. Lord J. *Sizes: the Illustrated Encyclopedia. How Big (or Little) Things Really Are.* New York: HarperPerennial; 1995.

3. Goldberg DP. *Manual of the General Health Questionnaire.* Windsor, Berks: NFER; 1978.

4. Peters WS. *Counting for Something: Statistical Principles and Personalities.* New York: Springer Verlag; 1987.

5. Arbuthnot J. An argument for divine providence, taken from the constant regularity observed in the births of both sexes. *Philosophical Transactions of the Royal Society.* 1710;27:186-190.

6. Everitt BS. *Chance Rules: an Informal Guide to Probability, Risk, and Statistics.* 2nd ed. New York: Springer; 2008.

7. Micceri T. The unicorn, the normal curve, and other improbable creatures. *Psychological Bulletin.* 1989;105:156-166.

8. Carstairs J, Shores E, Myors B. Australian norms and retest data for the Rey Auditory and Verbal Learning Test. *Australian Psychologist.* 2012;86:42-44.

)

CHAPTER **3**

DESCRIPTIVE STATISTICS

There are three types of lies: lies, damned lies and statistics!
ORIGIN UNCERTAIN

OBJECTIVES

After carefully reading this chapter you will know how to:

- recognise some possible statistical tricks or even 'lies'
- recognise statistical truth
- tell these apart
- describe reality so well that you and the people you communicate with can fully understand it, and gain something valuable from this understanding.

Introduction

Statistical methods can be seen as a series of tools that can aid the description and extrapolation of information. As such, they can be as conveniently divided into two categories, as can many other things in general and human nature. Descriptive statistics allows us to digest raw information that might otherwise give us and others information indigestion, and to present this information in a structured and useful manner. Inferential statistics allows us to extrapolate information from samples to populations, and to make inferences from the known to the unknown. You will be introduced to probability and to inferential statistics in Chapters 4 and 5, and to descriptive statistics in this one.

In 1954 a former editor of *Better Homes and Gardens* named Darrell Huff (1913–2001) wrote the world's first, and at this stage possibly *only*, statistics best seller. *How to Lie with Statistics* is a wonderful book with a wonderful title; it is still in print and has been translated into many languages.[1] This book was not written as a statistical textbook, or even as a primer for people who would like to increase their ability to be profitably dishonest, as perhaps was Machiavelli's sixteenth-century political manual, *The Prince*. *How to Lie with Statistics* was actually written to help people recognise the statistical truth by showing them how to recognise statistical untruth.

Descriptive statistics allows us to understand and perpetuate both information and disinformation, and this chapter will help you recognise the difference. Descriptive statistics when used wisely can even help us to navigate through information superhighway chaos by increasing our understanding of information and its vehicles of expression.

The purpose of descriptive statistics

A good place to begin our foray into descriptive statistics as a set of vital statistical building blocks is with the recognition that its purpose is to give us useful information, by describing and summarising data. Although many of us may not (yet) love statistics, many of us do love information. This is why gossip columns, pub trivia nights and the media are popular. Descriptive statistics allows us to process large amounts of data rapidly, by providing us with summary scores such as the mean, median and mode, and measures of how greatly individual scores vary from the summary score (standard deviation in the case of the mean). Descriptive statistics can also give us highly informative pictorial representations even of complex data, such as the graph and the plot. Descriptive statistics therefore allows us to both easily summarise and picture a thousand words, and more.

Norman and Streiner classically described the purpose of descriptive statistics as being to help us communicate results without trying to generalise beyond the sample that they came from to any other group.[2] To optimally communicate the results of a survey, study or experiment, it is generally useful to summarise data — for example, as mean illness severity — by utilising descriptive methods such as the mean (the sum of the measurements divided by the total number of measurements), the median (the middle value) and the mode (the most frequent value). Alternatively, we might valuably use tables to show frequencies such as occurrences of particular illnesses, which could be plotted across other categories such as seasons. These descriptive frequencies can be represented in tables that can include combinations of data (cross-tabulations) — for example, frequency of impulsive suicide attempts (or marriage proposals) combined with level of intoxication.

Descriptive statistics involves the interpretation, description and/or summarising of data, rather than simple enumeration, which involves merely reporting the counts of things, or 'headcounting', which in itself is not often particularly informative, unless you are a professional head-hunter. The medieval Domesday (or Doomsday) Book (Box 3.1) is an example of simple enumeration — counting heads or noses for the sake of counting heads or noses, or even to provide suitable employment for people who might otherwise not count. We modern information-rich people tend to dismiss such tallies as being mathematically primitive, but we habitually count and classify our CDs or socks or books, and often find the results highly useful.

Box 3.1 **Some interesting examples of nose counting**

When the early census known as the Domesday Book was compiled (the word *dome* in Middle English meant 'judgment'), the Normans had recently conquered England. Like many CEOs taking over a new outfit, they wanted to see exactly what they had acquired. The modern version of this early nose-counting census, however, is an application of statistics, in that it involves interpretation.

Further examples of simple nose counting can be seen in televised Australian Rules football matches, and undoubtedly also in gridiron, rugby, soccer, boxing and even, or perhaps especially, roller derbies. Sports 'statisticians' often earnestly and scrupulously count and report the raw number of kicks per quarter or punches per head of population, but do not usually attempt to calculate possibly much more meaningful information, such as the average time between the kicking of goals and behinds, or even their broader social significance.

Measures of central tendency

Things tend to even out over time. It is perhaps a happy tendency of many phenomena of nature, including human nature, that no matter how extreme a series of events, if there are enough of them over a long enough period they tend to become normally distributed. Measures of central tendency provide us with summaries of sets of scores that can be useful in that they give us a sense of the nature of many scores that are contained within a single score. The general principle underlying measures of central tendency is that things are rarely as bad (or as good) as they seem, and these measures can provide us with one or two measures that take the overall picture of a group of scores into account. A normal distribution of scores can, for example, be described in terms of its mean and standard deviation. Describing data in terms of measures of central tendency can provide us with a middle path between the high and low values contained in a data set.

There are different measures of central tendency that can provide us with summary information, just as there are different paths to peace, and each has its advantages and disadvantages. Which measure of central tendency we should apply depends on the nature of our particular information situation.

The mean

The most commonly used type of average is the arithmetic mean, which is generally known to the layperson simply as the average. Laypeople may sometimes be derided by more technically advanced people for their lack of technique, but it may be useful to remember that few experts in any area were born experts, and that many excellent ideas have been hatched by laypeople. It may also be useful to bear in mind that the truly average, like the truly perfect, is usually just an ideal. Nobody really has 2.3 cars, or 0.4 of a dog or 0.0001 of a pet snake.

The formula for calculating the arithmetic mean is:

$$\text{Mean} = \frac{\sum x}{N}$$

This can be translated into English as:

The mean is the sum of all of your scores, divided by how many scores you have.

An ecologically valid health-science–related example of calculating the mean can be found in a hypothetical scenario in which a surgeon, a nurse, a health administrator, a dentist, a psychologist, a radiographer, a general practitioner, a physiotherapist, a biostatistician and a vet all go out to lunch. Perhaps the new health administrator wants to meet a broad selection of staff, or perhaps this is just a fairly low-probability random occurrence. The lunch bill comes to $220, which means that the mean meal cost is $220 (sum of meal cost scores) divided by 10 (number, N, of diners), which is $22 a head (or nose). This is all perfectly simple and clear so far, but as with most good stories there is a perhaps unexpected plot twist lurking here, which could force us to think carefully about what type of measure of central tendency is most appropriate to our situation.

What happens if we have extreme values? What happens in our statistical training restaurant if 9 of its health-science customers settled for the house special, baked beans on toast, and a glass of house wine for a total of $15 each, and one of the diners (you might like to guess which) ordered out-of-season asparagus, lobster surprise and imported champagne for a total of $85? Would you be happy to split your share of the bill on the basis of the arithmetic mean as the 'average' meal price? This is actually a common statistical practice, often applied by people who are not skilled statisticians, and it certainly seems fair, but is it always? In this situation our average price is $15 + $15 + $15 + $15 + $15 + $15 + $15 + $15 + $15 + $85 = $220, divided by our N of 10 = $22, but the last individual bill score is far higher than 9 of the 10 other scores. It could therefore be reasonably argued by any of the 9 non-lobster-ordering diners that the mean has given us an inflated single summary score of our data. We may therefore consider using an alternative measure of central tendency that is less sensitive to extreme scores (or changing our restaurant ordering practices, or job).

The median

In situations where very high and very low scores can distort the arithmetic mean, it is often useful to use the median measure of central tendency instead. The medium point in a ranked distribution of scores is the median. The median is like a dear friend who is totally unfazed by everything we do, perhaps because they have stopped listening to us, and are therefore comfortably immune to our highs and lows. The median is the point at which half the scores in a distribution are higher, and half the scores are lower. The median, then, can be seen as the statistical middle ground, the perfect balance.

The formulas for working out medians are refreshingly simple and we can present them in English without having first presented them in algebraic. The formula for working out the median when there are an odd number of scores (when there are no tied observations) is:

The median is the middle score.

The formula for working out the median when there is an even number of scores (when there are tied observations) is:

The median is the first middle score plus the second middle score divided by two.

We can provide a variant of our ongoing restaurant example that illustrates the calculation of the median. There are 10 individual meal costs for our 10 diners, which is an even number, which means that we need to employ the even number median formula. This results in the median score being the sum of the middle two individual meal order scores, $15 + $15 = $30, divided by 2 = $15. In this case, therefore, the median of $15 is a far more sensible reflection of our individual scores than is the mean of $22, because it more closely resembles the majority of the scores (meal prices). If we take any five of our meal price scores, we can calculate the median by using the median formula for an odd number of scores. The middle score, or median, will also be $15.

House-price data provide a common general illustration of how the median can be less sensitive to the vicissitudes of extreme scores than is the mean, and these are usually given as median values rather than as mean values for exactly this reason. To provide a tenuously health-science–related example of the appropriate summarisation of house-price data, what if one of the five houses sold in the last 12 months in the Health Heights Hospital Estate sold for $220,000 because it had storm damage, while the other four each sold for $320,000? Is the median price of $320,000 a better measure of central tendency in this case than the arithmetic mean price of $300,000? Our perceptions of the relative equity of the median or mean may depend on whether we are the one with the lobster or the storm-damaged house, but the general principle to be noted here is that we need to choose our measures of central tendency wisely.

Measures of central tendency can have too little as well as too much sensitivity to the variability of scores, and the median scores in the above examples of $15 and $320,000 do not tell us much about what is happening in the groups of numbers from which these medians were calculated. A compromise between the advantages and disadvantages of the mean and the median is the trimmed mean.[3] This involves removing the top and bottom 10% or 5% of the scores and then taking the mean of the rest. In this way the statistic protects us against extreme scores (such as lobster lunch prices) but tries to take more of the scores into account than does the median, which could be termed a 50% trimmed mean. The trimmed mean should be used more often than it is, because it reduces the effect of eccentrically high or low scores, but otherwise utilises more information in the data than does the median, which ignores most of what is going on, like a friend you have known too long.

The mode

The mode is simply the score in a distribution of scores that occurs most often. If a group of 10 health scientists or students of health sciences go out to lunch and five of them have lobster surprise (possibly because they have just received a large research grant), four of them have baked beans on toast, and one has nothing at all, then the lobsters are the mode. In a series of events, the mode is the most common. Given that the famous and influential *Mode* magazine might not like to be associated with the word 'common', a more appropriate definition might be the most 'usual' event or better yet, the most 'popular' event.

Measures of dispersion

In life, and in its research and clinical empirical measurement, we are often interested in how far scores and groups of scores vary from their mean, so it is important for us to be able to calculate measures of dispersion. In IQ testing, for example, we will not know the full meaning of a score unless we can compare the distance between this score and the IQ mean with the general distance between IQ scores and the mean. An IQ score of 112, for example, means that this score is 12 points away from the IQ mean, but unless we have an average distance from the mean we do not know whether this distance is large or small. Measures of dispersion therefore tell us to what extent scores in a group of scores vary around their measure of central tendency, and what the average of this variance is.

The variance

The variance is a measure of dispersion of a group of scores from their mean and provides important information on the amount of variation of the values of a variable. The variance is commonly used in several statistical procedures that will be discussed in later chapters, and we calculate it by first summing the squared values of the differences between each score and their mean. The square of each difference is used so that all the numbers are positive. If we used unsquared scores, they would sum to zero (because negative and positive numbers cancel each other out when summed) and we would not have a measure of dispersion.

The formula for working out the variance is:

$$S^2 = \frac{\sum (x - \bar{x})^2}{N-1}$$

Particularly when we are dealing with small samples, it is better to use N − 1 than N. This is because, for mathematical reasons that are not at all essential to our thickening plot, this gives us a more accurate estimate. This formula can be translated into English as:

The variance is the sum of the squared differences (deviations) between each of your scores and their mean, divided by the number of scores (N) minus one.

An example of calculating the variance that relates to our restaurant example is as follows: five health-science professionals and students go into a restaurant to celebrate getting a research grant; one orders baked beans on toast for $15, three order lobster surprise at $65 per head (the successful research grant team) and one orders nothing at all (the unsuccessful research team). The mean is therefore $15 + $65 + $65 + $65 + $0 divided by 5 = $42. The group is now getting a group discount on the lobster surprise meal deal, which has been suitably calculated by the statistically savvy restaurant manager. The variance of meal price scores can be calculated by summing the squared difference of each individual score from the mean, which is $27^2 + $23^2 + $23^2 + $23^2 + $42^2 = $4080 divided by N − 1 (which is 5 − 1), so our variance is $1020.

The standard deviation

The standard deviation is the square root of the variance, and this can be seen as the average abnormality. In other words, it is the average distance from the mean, or the average variance, which is used in several statistical tests that will be described in later chapters, and referred to in tables of the normal distribution (a tale of two tails).

The formula for working out the standard deviation is:

$$S = \sqrt{\text{Variance}}$$

This can be translated into English as:

The standard deviation is the square root of the variance.

The World Health Organization provides publicly available world health data that we can use in a real health-related example of calculating standard deviation.[4] If we take the life expectancy at birth figures for 15 countries, and do not adjust for the different population sizes of these 15 countries (which we would, or at least should, normally do), then based on the data provided in Table 3.1 we can calculate a mean of 70.73, and a standard deviation of 11.80. The sum of the squared differences from the mean is 1948.75. Dividing this by N − 1 (14) = 139.20, which is the variance. The square root of the variance gives us the standard deviation — the average variance from the mean — which is 11.80. We square and then square root our values, so that the sum of the positive and negative differences from the mean do not equal zero.

Our best guesses of the specific values of the underlying mean and the standard deviation of the population from which our sample has been drawn are simply the sample mean and the sample standard deviation. This is called 'point estimation', the estimation of a single point, such as the population mean. Unfortunately, if our sample is small, it will not be a very good guess, and the use of different samples may give us different results. Characteristics of samples will be covered in more detail

TABLE 3.1 LIFE EXPECTANCY AT BIRTH DATA, 2009, FOR 15 COUNTRIES, MALES AND FEMALES COMBINED

Country	Life expectancy		
	x	$x - $ mean	$(x - $ mean$)^2$
Afghanistan	48	−22.73	516.65
Australia	82	11.27	127.01
Canada	81	10.27	105.47
China	74	3.27	10.69
Germany	80	9.27	85.93
India	65	−5.73	32.83
Indonesia	68	−2.73	7.45
Japan	83	12.27	150.55
Kenya	60	−10.63	112.99
New Zealand	81	−10.27	105.47
Papua New Guinea	63	−7.73	59.75
Russia	68	−2.73	7.45
UK	80	9.27	85.93
USA	79	8.27	68.39
Zimbabwe	49	21.73	472.19

Mean = 70.73 Σx^2 = 1948.75

in Chapter 5, but do not worry because there are answers to most problems, even statistical ones, and as a former prime minister of Australia, Malcolm Fraser, once famously remarked, 'Life wasn't meant to be easy'!

Graphs and plots

It has been wisely written by an ancient Chinese descriptive statistician that a picture is worth a thousand words. We tend to find it easier to understand complex information when it is presented in some kind of pictorial form, such as in a graph or plot. This phenomenon was recognised by the inventors of the widely used contemporary computing systems that allow us to click onto a visual icon rather than having to type out our computer instructions in words. The power of representing information visually as graphs and plots is also employed in descriptive statistics, which includes graphical representations of information. Graphical methods of displaying information, such as the histogram, bar chart, pie chart and box and whisker plot, are widely used in the health sciences.

The histogram and the bar chart

Histograms graphically display distributions of continuous data, such as temperatures or height reached, and generally have no space between their bars. The great English statistician Karl Pearson coined the term 'histogram' in 1891 in a lecture that he gave on maps and chartograms. (Pearson's contribution will be discussed more fully in the section on Pearson's correlation in Chapter 9.) Bar charts graphically represent discrete data, such as percentage of gross domestic product (GDP) spent annually on healthcare, and generally have a space between their bars. Both bar charts and histograms present the divisions of scores on the *x*-axis (horizontal axis) of a graph and the number (frequency) or percentage of each score on the *y*-axis (vertical axis).

A general example of the histogram in action relates to people's heights, which are typically measured on continuous scales such as centimetres and typically form normal distributions. A distribution of human heights plotted on a frequency histogram is shown in Figure 3.1. You may notice that this distribution is probably of the heights of a single gender (just males or just females) because it is not bimodal (that is, there are different characteristics for males and females). You may also notice that this

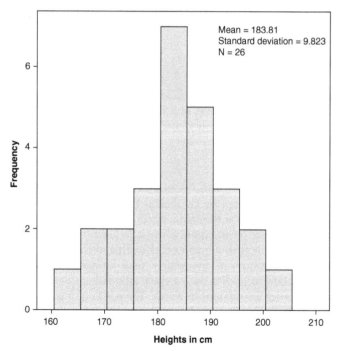

Fig 3.1 A frequency histogram of human heights in centimetres

distribution is probably of male heights because of the magnitude of its values.

A health-related example of the bar chart in action can be constructed using publicly available data from the US Department of Health and Human Services, National Center for Health Statistics.[5] Figure 3.2 shows health expenditure for the year 2007 as a percentage of GDP for seven OECD countries. The data can be presented in textual form alphabetically as: Australia, 8.9%; Canada, 10.1%; France, 11.0%; Korea, 6.3%; Mexico, 5.9%; UK, 8.4%; USA, 16.0%. The data can also be presented alphabetically as in the bar chart shown in Figure 3.2. We leave it to you to decide which form of information presentation is easier to interpret.

The pie chart

The pie chart is named after the food that it resembles and is conveniently structured into sections that correspond to pie slices, where the size of each slice is proportional to the quantity of data that it represents. The pie chart was probably first used in 1801, in the *Statistical Breviary*, by William Playfair (1759–1823).[6] It is a useful way of presenting information, especially information regarding proportions, because it is particularly easy to understand and digest. It is therefore perhaps the most commonly used descriptive statistic by business and the popular media, but it has been discouraged for serious applications by some statistical

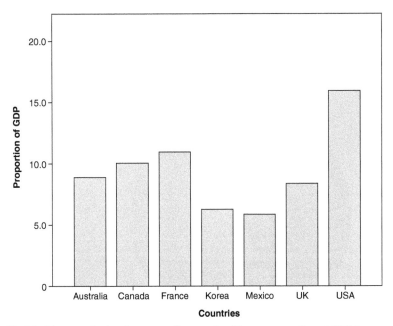

Fig 3.2 **A bar graph showing expenditure on health as a proportion of GDP for seven OECD countries**

experts. This is because comparisons of slices of the information pie with one another and with other pies can be indirect. The pie chart is best used, therefore, for comparing individual information slices of pie with their entire information pie. It also needs to be remembered that the pie chart is appropriate for use with nominal data, but not with continuous data.

It is natural for us to recognise comparative proportions of information within a pie chart as smaller or larger slices of a pie. This potentially useful descriptive statistic can therefore be regarded as the opposite of pie in the sky and more like apple pie, in that it is friendly, appealing and easy to understand. It could even be said that pie charts provide a useful bridge between our everyday lives and our statistical lives because they look like what they are and can readily convey any type of information in an intuitively meaningful manner.

A health-science example of the pie chart in action can again be constructed using US Department of Health and Human Services data. Figure 3.3 shows the comparative sizes of the 2008 US health-budget pie, in terms of percentage of expenditure on different facets of health. This information can also be represented textually in alphabetical order as: hospital care, 30.7%; nursing home care, 5.8%; other, 32.3%; physician and clinical services, 21.2%; prescription drugs, 10.0%. We will again leave you to decide which form of information presentation is easier to interpret.

Perhaps interestingly, the data contained in Figure 3.3 reveals that 10.0% of the 2008 US health budget (which was approximately US$2.3 trillion) was spent on prescription drugs. This means that approximately

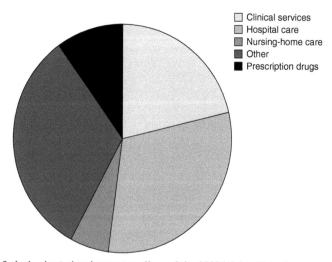

Fig 3.3 **A pie chart showing sector slices of the 2008 US health budget**

230 billion government dollars were spent in the US alone in 2008 on prescription drugs, which might explain why there is considerable research undertaken internationally into the efficacy of current and potential drugs. Perhaps also interestingly, 5.9% of the 2008 US health budget was spent on nursing-home care, which means that approximately 135 billion government dollars were spent in the US alone on nursing-home care, which might explain why there is considerable research undertaken internationally into positive ageing. These are particularly noteworthy data when we consider that international population forecasts suggest that by the year 2050 the world population of people above the age of 65 years will almost triple, from 6.9% in 2000, to 19.3%.

Box 3.2 **Pie in the sky?**

Peripherally related to the pie chart is the pie index, which has just been devised for your descriptive statistical education and entertainment. The pie index provides a useful, if informal, index of inflation. In 1970 a meat pie cost about 14 cents in Australia, or 16 cents with sauce. In 2010 a meat pie cost about $4 in Australia, or slightly over $3 in Seattle, where you can get Australian meat pies shipped to you anywhere in the world in quantities of 12 or more.

The pie inflation index tells us how much things cost now compared with what they cost 40 years ago in relation to meat pies. This index therefore provides a proportional indication of whether particular goods or services are dearer or cheaper than they once were, comparative to a goods and service constant (the pie).

In 1970 the median house price in Australia was about $15,000, which was then the cost of about 10,700 pies. In 2010 the median house price in Australia was about $430,000, which was then the cost of about 107,500 pies. Australian house prices could therefore be said to have risen roughly tenfold between 1970 and 2010 comparative to a constant consuming cost (of pies).

In 1970 the cheapest price for a return flight to Europe from Australia was about $1500, or about 10,700 pies. In 2010 the cheapest price for a return ticket to Europe from Australia was about $1500, or 375 pies. Australia to Europe airfares could therefore be said to have fallen almost thirtyfold between 1970 and 2010 comparative to a constant consuming cost (of pies).

The meat pie was very incidentally once described by a former premier of New South Wales (and later Australian Minister for Foreign Affairs), Bob Carr, as 'Australia's national dish'.

Box plot

The box plot, otherwise know as the box and whisker plot, can provide us with a useful summary of the range of our data, including between our smallest data value (observation) and the largest data value. This plot also describes data in terms of how much is contained within various divisions, such as into 3 tertiles, 4 quartiles, 5 quintiles or even 10 deciles. Box plots can also be used to show us the points between which the percentage of data that interest us fall. The spacings between the different parts of the components of a box plot, or box and whiskers plot, can show us the degree of dispersion of our data, whether it is skewed (see Chapter 2), and whether there are outliers.

The lower and upper boundaries of the box in a box plot always represent the 25th and 75th percentiles and are the points below which 25% and 75% of our data fall. The middle line of a box plot is always the median, or 50th percentile, the point below which half of our data falls. The whiskers of a box and whisker plot can be used to show us the highest and lowest data points, or the number of data points up to the highest and lowest tertiles (divided into 3), quartiles (4), quintiles (5) or even deciles (10).

A general example of a box and whisker plot is shown in Figure 3.4, which is a box and whisker plot of the height data that we previously displayed as a frequency histogram.

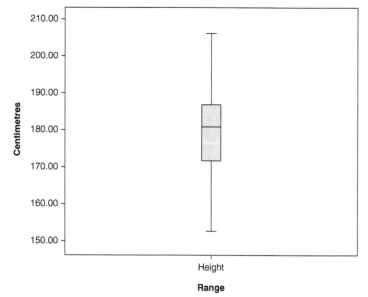

Fig 3.4 **A box and whisker plot of male human height data**

How to recognise descriptive statistical untruths

It is now time to introduce you to some basic descriptive statistical abuses that are commonly perpetuated by advertisers, including scientific advertisers, to 'black-magically' transform information into disinformation. This is typically accomplished by distorting facts either deliberately (statistical deceit) or accidentally (statistical ignorance), and it can have diabolical consequences if not recognised by either the information receiver or the information transceiver. This section therefore corresponds to the Hogwarts' 'Defence against the Dark Arts' courses described in the *Harry Potter* book and movie series.

Misleading levels of accuracy

It is common for advertisers and other applied disinformation theorists to bombard us with 'statistics' such as that product X or drug Y will make our hair or our patients' hair 68.34% stronger, or reduce their rash by 414.29%. Health scientists applying for grants are often just as aware as advertisers that it sounds far more convincing to ask for three million, two hundred and two dollars to fund a research program than it does to ask for exactly three million dollars or even for 'a lot of money'. People quoting trade or professional repair jobs to us often employ this information enhancement principle, and appear to have either been taught or innately acquired the knowledge that their customers are even more likely to take seriously an outrageous quote of $302.75, or better still $297.25, to fix their plumbing or tooth filling than they are to accept a quote of exactly $300. Statistical malpractices such as misleading levels of inaccuracy can also distract us from asking such basic statistically literate questions as '68.34% stronger than what?'.

Misleading graphs

There is a reason why information presentations such as stories or graphs are best started at the beginning, and this is that if you start them anywhere else they tend to confuse and confound rather than to explain. If we see a graph starting at zero showing that patient satisfaction levels in our local hospital have increased by 2.2% in the last year from 41.2% to 43.4% (Fig 3.5), this relatively steady information is unlikely to cause us unbridled satisfaction, if we have a professional or personal desire for a considerable improvement in patient satisfaction. If we see the same information in a graph starting at 40% (Fig 3.6), this might cause us considerable and inappropriate satisfaction — as long as we do not look at it closely or think carefully about it. This is due to the statistically misrepresented fact that, if a graph starts at 40, 43.4% looks much larger than 41.2%. Graphs, like life, actually properly begin at 0, and not 40.

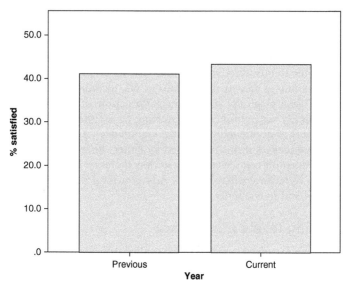

Fig 3.5 **A bar graph showing the percentage of patient satisfaction with hospital treatment, with the y axis commencing at 0%**

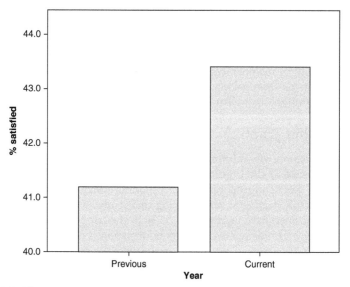

Fig 3.6 **A bar graph showing the percentage of patient satisfaction with hospital treatment, with the y axis commencing at 40%**

Misleading numbers

We all know that 99% fat free sounds a lot better than 1% fat does. This illustrates the phenomenon that the same information can be represented in many different ways, some of which make it look good, some of which make it look bad. Advertisers, accountants, advocates and media workers tend to be experts at putting their desired spin on their information offerings, which can transform it into disinformation. This is why basic statistical literacy will help to protect us from the information intrigues of the disinformation pushers, and prevent us from joining them.

We can make a number sound bad by saying that the average annual income in a suburb that we do not like is 'less than $49,000 a year' and by saying that the average annual income in a suburb that we do like is 'more than $48,000 a year'. Information disseminators can be divided in the same way as magic disseminators can — into black and white ones. Black magic has been defined as magic practised for oneself, while white magic has been defined as magic practised for others. The same standards could usefully be applied to statistics. Perhaps if you are ever in a position of having to sell a project or a product that nobody but you can see the value of, you could forget the above advice, just once, and try something like 'Diet Lard, 1% fat free!'.

Incomplete data

It is amazing how easy it is to lie statistically, or at least to fail to tell the truth, the *whole* truth and nothing but the truth — without actually lying. This can be accomplished simply by leaving out important information. An example of this practice is the statistics that were presented a few years ago showing that American soldiers stationed in Iraq in the first Gulf War had a lower death rate there than they did at home. These descriptive statistics told the truth, but not the whole truth, because they left out the rest of the story — that most of the American soldiers serving in Iraq were young and often black or Hispanic — and tended to come from cities that had high murder rates, especially of young blacks and Hispanics. It may be true to state that some Americans were safer in the Iraq war than they were at home, but this should be seen in the light of the complete data picture, which reveals more about the safety of some American cities than it does about the safety of being a soldier in Iraq.

Another health-related example of the disinformation dangers of using incomplete data is the often reported statistics that apparently reveal that we are safer travelling in large cars than in small ones. Such statistics are popular with the manufacturers of large cars, and their advertisers, especially when faced with a decrease in large-car sales due to the increasing cost of traditional fuels. Large-car safety statistics have been around, however, for almost as long as large cars have been around. A study reported by *Time Magazine* in 1964 presented some 'sober statistics' about the comparative safety of driving in large cars,[7] but it neglected to complete the descriptive statistical picture by mentioning that the reports cited also stated that people who drive in small cars were less likely to be in accidents, so the overall accident risk of drivers of large and small cars was about the same. The same principle applies to asking questions of descriptive statistics as to asking questions of any source of information — commonsense.

Conclusion

Descriptive statistics describe information, and what separates information wheat from information chaff is whether it is described precisely, appropriately and honestly. In the next chapter we will introduce you to probability, for its own sake and as a prelude to its use in inferential statistics. If you liked, or at least respected, the usefulness of descriptive statistics, then you will love, or at least admire, the usefulness of inferential statistics.

Quick reference summary

- Descriptive statistics allows us to digest raw information that might otherwise give us and others information indigestion, and to present this information in a structured and useful manner.

- Descriptive statistics involves the interpretation, description and/or summarising of data, rather than simple enumeration, which involves merely reporting the counts of things, or 'headcounting'.

- Descriptive measures of central tendency provide us with summaries of scores that describe many scores in a single score. These include the mean (average) score, the median (middle score) and the mode (most common score).

- In life and its research, we are often interested in how much scores vary from their mean, so we need to be able to calculate measures of dispersion. These include the variance (of scores from the mean) and the standard deviation (average variance).

- Descriptive statistics includes the powerful visual representation of information as graphs and plots, which include the histogram, the bar chart, the pie chart and the box and whisker plot.

- It is easy to use descriptive statistics to lie, or at least to avoid portraying the complete information truth. Examples of the descriptive statistical dark arts to look out for (but not resort to) include not starting a graph at zero, and not giving the complete information story.

References

1. Huff D. *How to Lie with Statistics*. Illust. I. Geis. New York: Norton; 1954.

2. Norman GR, Streiner DL. *PDQ Statistics*. 3rd ed. Hamilton, Ontario: BC Decker; 2003.

3. Wilcox RR. *Introduction to Robust Estimation and Hypothesis Testing*. 2nd ed. Boston: Elsevier; 2005.

4. World health Organization. *World Health Statistics 2011*. Available online at <http://www.who.int/gho/publications/world_health_statistics/EN_WHS2011_Full.pdf>. Accessed 21 Sept 2012.

5. US Department of health and Human Services. *Health, United States, 20120, with Special Feature on Death and Dying*. Available online at <http://www.cdc.gov/nchs/data/hus/hus10.pdf#122>. Accessed 21 Sept 2012.

6. Friendly M. The golden age of statistical graphics. *Statistical Science*. 2008;23(4):502-535.

7. *Time Magazine*, 12 June 1964.

CHAPTER 4

PROBABILITY

The probable is what usually happens.

ARISTOTLE (384–322 BC)

OBJECTIVES

After carefully reading this chapter you will know the:

- importance of probability, in statistics and in life

- workings and underlying principles of some basic probability rules

- nature of probability distributions and how they relate to the calculation of probability

- cure for uncertainty.

Introduction

Apart from statistics, what other extremely popular, well-paid and glamorous activity is largely based on the laws of probability? The answer is gambling, which can be even more of a process of playing the odds than life is. Like many statistical tools, probability theory was developed to meet particular needs, and these needs historically included those of gamblers to improve their chances of winning, or at least better understand why they were losing.

We live in an extremely uncertain world, and probably always did. In our early human days there was considerable uncertainty and this could cause us considerable stress if we did not deal with it optimally. These early stresses included some fairly straightforward challenging life situations, such as not knowing the whereabouts of our next meal or a sabre-toothed tiger, or whether we might end up providing rather than receiving the next meal. Sabre-toothed tigers are, incidentally, traditionally used as examples of ecological validity in a range of health-science disciplines, so we have now met our sabre-toothed tiger quota. We can also meet our quota for references to the popular modern philosopher Eckhart Tolle by mentioning his notion that uncertainty is a profound cause of human unhappiness, and that the antidote for this is changing our attitude towards it.

Our modern uncertainties usually do not involve survival, but, in terms of Maslow's hierarchy of needs, our growing information saturation can make achieving our higher life needs such as fulfilment more uncertain.[1] Understanding something about probability and how it relates to our daily life may therefore help us recognise that uncertainty — like life, like statistics — is inherently harmless and often enjoyable.

Probability and statistics

Probability is a key concept in statistics and in life. Whether we realise it or not, we are all (usually unpaid) probability theorists. Every day of our lives we make decisions, big and small. Should I have bacon and eggs for breakfast, or muesli and fruit? Should I take the train to work, or drive my car, or ride my bike? Who should I marry and how many guests should we invite to the wedding? We use probability to answer life's questions, and how successful we are in life often depends on how well we play its odds. We do not live in a random universe, as Einstein pointed out, but we do live in an often uncertain one.

We live in a universe governed by perfectly sensible rules and regulations known as natural laws, but unfortunately these are often only perfectly sensible and natural to the extent that we can understand and predict them. Life as we know it would be something other than life as we know it if we knew all of the answers or even all of the questions — if we had 100% certainty. Our life decisions often require us to hypothesise a best guess as to what we expect to happen if we act in a certain way, with varying levels of associated certainty. What we eat for breakfast, how we get to work and which jobs we arrive at are based on decisions that are determined by our (usually informal) calculations of the relative chances of success of each of our options.

Our life hypotheses and their informal probability testing provide a familiar and useful conceptual basis for our understanding of statistical probability. Inferential statistics will be covered in more detail in Chapter 5, but it basically involves inferring characteristics of populations on the basis of observed characteristics of samples — generalising from the known to the unknown.

We frequently use samples of our life experiences to generalise with a level of uncertainty that is acceptable to us. If we have three bad food experiences in a restaurant, we may generalise that this place is not good for our health, and not return to it. We may not realise it, but this action is based on our personal level of required certainty for our generalisation to be correct. Probability is therefore not merely a useful inferential statistical construct, but a specialised extension of a real-life one. Using probability theory in inferential statistics to compare the efficacy of a range of clinical treatments based on our samples, for example, is an extension of using an informal probability analysis to compare the efficacy of a range of restaurants, based on our samples.

Applied probability theory

Some elementary probability rules and underlying principles will now be presented in the context of descriptions of some general applications of probability.

Coin tossing

Introductory texts on computer programming often offer an elementary programming example that ends up with the words 'Hello World!' displayed on the computer screen. In the teaching of probability theory there is also a venerable tradition, that of using examples that involve the tossing of coins, and we will respectfully continue this conceptually useful, as well as venerable, tradition here. Coin tossing is not a particularly glamorous example of the principles of probability, compared with life and gambling examples, and James Bond probably never did it. Coin tossing is, however, now practised legally in some Australian casinos, where two coins are tossed in a game somewhat unimaginatively known as 'two-up'.[2,3] Perhaps unfortunately, discussions of probability have traditionally focused on the tossing of only a single coin, until now.

If we randomly throw a coin in the air, the probability of it coming down with either heads or tails facing up is exactly half — if we discount such wildly unlikely eventualities as the possibility it may land on its edge, or disappear into a previously unsuspected dimension, or be eaten by a homework-eating dog. This value, then, is the statistical probability of the event, which is 0.50 in this case, or 50%. There is a simple rule for calculating the probability of a single event that shows us why this is so:

$$\text{Probability A} = \frac{\text{number of favourable outcomes}}{\text{number of possible outcomes}}$$

The favourable outcome in this case is the coin landing with either heads or tails facing up, depending on which we have called. There is one favourable outcome (heads or tails) and two possible outcomes (heads or tails) so the probability value here is 1 ÷ 2 = 0.50, or 50%.

If we are interested in the probability of any one of a set of mutually exclusive events occurring, then the probability of the event occurring can be calculated by using the additive probability rule, which is used to calculate the sum of the events' separate probabilities:

$$\text{Probability A or B} \ldots = \text{probability of A} + \text{B} \ldots$$

Therefore if the probability of a coin coming up heads is 0.50 and the probability of it coming up tails is 0.50, then the probability of it coming up either heads or tails is 1.0.

If we throw a coin in the air twice or if we throw up two coins once, things get more interesting, or at least more complicated. Our chance of achieving two heads is now half as likely as achieving a heads result when we toss one coin, which means a 25% chance or a probability of 0.25. Chances are that you have noticed that there is a pattern emerging here, and this pattern can be formally described. If two events A and B are independent, then the probability of them both happening can be calculated by using the multiplicative rule:

$$\text{Probability (A} + \text{B)} = \text{Probability A} \times \text{Probability B}$$

Given that a fair coin has a probability of 0.50 of coming up heads when we throw it, the probability of two coin tosses (such as in a game of two-up) both coming up heads is therefore 0.50 × 0.50 = 0.25, or 25%. Similarly, the chances of three coin tosses all coming up heads (or all tails) is 0.50 × 0.50 × 0.50 = 0.125, or 12.5%. This may sound fairly technical, probably because it is, but at least this calculation is straightforward and can be applied to more complex examples.

If we toss a coin n times then the probability of there being n heads, or n tails, or of any one specified pattern of heads and tails is equal to 1 ÷ (2 to the power of n). The probability of throwing 3 heads in a row is therefore 1 ÷ 8, or 1 in 8 (0.125). The probability of throwing 10 heads

---

Box 4.1 **Pub trivia nights**

Probability rules tend to get more interesting when they are applied to real-life situations, so here is a real-life general example that certainly does not come from the 'random avenue, statistical city' genre of unrealistic data.

Pub trivia nights are a rich source of realistic examples of many life and statistical principles. There was an exercise in applied probability theory held every Wednesday night at a particular pub trivia evening that we once habitually frequented. Approximately 100 amateur probability theorists were systematically asked to put aside their bustling beer and brains for about 5 minutes, and stand up with their hands on either their heads or their tails. A coin was then tossed, and if the participants in the game guessed wrong, a 50% probability, they were required to sit down. The coin kept being tossed until there was only one person left standing, who won a jug of beer.

A question could then have been asked by anyone interested and sober enough to ask it: 'In order to win the jug of beer, the coin toss was correctly predicted n times, what is the probability of that occurring?' Interestingly, even in the midst of such significant numbers of potential applied probability practitioners, one occasionally heard comments such as 'It's come up three heads in a row — the next one has to be tails!' This seems to indicate a stronger belief in magic than in science, but humankind has often assigned illusory certainty to random situations.

---

in a row is $1 \div 1024$ or 1 in 1024, and the chance of 20 heads in a row is a little less than one in a million. Even after a run of 20 heads in a row, the chance of the next coin coming up heads is still 0.50. The probability of 21 heads in a row might be minuscule, but the chance of each coin coming up heads (or tails) remains at 0.50 — the coins have no memory.

Birth ratios

The ratio of male to female births involves another example of two events that are approximately equally likely, but they are actually not quite 50:50. This ratio illustrates an important consideration when applying the rules for calculating the probability of more than one independent event occurring — that the events have to be independent. If the

---

Box 4.2 **A noteworthy coin tosser**

There have been several noted coin tossers in statistical history, the most famous perhaps being the esteemed British statistician Karl (originally Carl) Pearson (1857–1936), who gave us the Pearson product moment correlation and the chi-square test, and coined the term 'standard deviation'. In 1900, some years before television was invented, Pearson tossed a coin 24,000 times and obtained 12,012 heads (0.5005). For a fair coin, the probability for each coin toss of coming up heads is 0.50, over an infinite series of tosses. You will learn more about Dr Pearson in later chapters.

---

probability of producing a boy is x, does this mean that the probability of producing 3 boys in a row is x by x by x? It may not, because these events (the birth of a boy or a girl) may not be independent. There is evidence that boys are more likely to be born early on in the marriage (for example, child 1 and child 2 are more likely to be boys), when marital contact is more likely to be vigorous and regular, while girls tend to be born later in the marriage (for example, child 3 and child 4 are more likely to be girls).[4] The conditions of being born either female or male may be related and therefore not independent, so it is inappropriate in such circumstances to apply the above rules.

Gambling

We can generalise the application of the above probability rules to calculate our chances of winning at various games in a casino, and we can use exactly the same principles to apply probability theory to the general and health-related examples that we will provide in subsequent chapters.

The longest winning series ever recorded at the famous roulette tables of Monte Carlo, Monaco, involved red coming up successively 28 times.[5,6] In roulette wheels that have one zero, the probability of a single red number coming up is 18 (total red numbers) divided by 37 (total numbers on a roulette wheel, including zero). The probability of the above sequence occurring is therefore (18 ÷ 37) to the power of 28, or (18 ÷ 37) × (18 ÷ 37) × (18 ÷ 37), and so on, to a total of 28 times. The odds are therefore approximately 578 million to one against red (or black) coming up 28 times in a row. Anyone who stayed on red for the entire 28 spins would have made a cool 578 million dollars for an outlay of one dollar. People being what and who we are, though, they almost certainly all rushed onto black after a series of spins coming up red, in the firm belief that the cosmic pendulum had to swing back again.

One of the many practical advantages of a basic understanding of probability theory is that it can help us to choose which games are most profitable to play in a casino, as well as to interpret the results of a wide range of health-science–related inferential statistics. The application of probability theory to gambling has a long history in statistics, and indeed probably originated (most likely in France) as a practical response to the desire of gamblers to better and more successfully understand their odds.

The probability of our winning at roulette depends on the number of zeroes there are on the roulette wheel. There are 36 numbers and a single zero on Australian, European and South American roulette wheels, and 36 numbers and two zeroes on most North American roulette wheels. Betting on one of 36 numbers appears to mean that we have one chance of winning and 35 ordinary chances of losing, and the gambling odds reflect this, because we will be paid $36 if our $1 bet wins. The fact that there is a zero at play, though, is what makes a casino a casino and not a fun parlour. A single zero means that we actually have one chance in 37 of winning, which gives the casino a profit of 1/37, or 2.70%. In casinos with two zeroes on their roulette wheels, the casino's profit is or 2/38, or 5.26%.

Winning back 97.30%, or even 94.74%, of every dollar that we bet in a casino is actually comparatively excellent odds, compared with other gambles. If we visit a casino somewhere other than North America and play only roulette, we will do as well financially as we would if we took one in 37 notes out of our purses or wallets and set fire to them. This is far better odds than if we played on a poker machine or bought a ticket in a lottery, which typically only give us back about $80 for every $100 that we spend — approximately equivalent to taking one note in five out of our purses or wallets and setting fire to them. Basic statistical literacy, therefore, can give us the highly useful practical power of being able to ask meaningful questions of any data such as how many tickets are there in the raffle, what is their selling price, what are the prizes worth and therefore how much of the ticket price is profit? Probability theory gives us a working knowledge of truth, whether the truth that we are interested in relates to gambling or to anything else.

Health sciences

A group of health researchers in the UK were interested in whether people's quality of life, as measured by control, autonomy, self-realisation and pleasure scores (CASP, a measure of generic quality of life), has an impact on their longevity. The researchers followed up 291 people whose quality-of-life profiles had been recorded via the British Household Panel Survey, and found that in the 5-year follow-up period the probability of mortality from all causes for a high-quality-of-life-scoring group was approximately double that of a low-quality-of-life-scoring group.[7] Good quality of life can therefore help us to live longer as well as help to make living longer worthwhile, and there are many factors that can potentially increase or decrease our probability of high life quality. To link two of our applied probability examples, gambling (as you would probably expect) decreases the probability of a high quality of life.[8]

Box 4.3 **Probability and the games people play**

The most visited square in Monopoly is the Jail square,[9] and the least visited is, perhaps appropriately, Chance. The most visited property in the standard US Monopoly game is Illinois Avenue, which corresponds to Trafalgar Square in the UK version. The least visited property in the American game is Mediterranean Avenue, which corresponds to Old Kent Road in the UK version. That might explain why rent is so cheap there — $2 in the 1960s Australian version of the UK game. Our progress in games such as these is based on the probability of certain results, and people who understand such probabilities tend to do well at such games.

There is a game called Pass the Pigs® that illustrates probability well, if idiosyncratically. Freddie Wong, incidentally, has a web page entirely devoted to Milton Bradley's statistically informative tossing plastic pigs game (http://passpigs.tripod.com/), which has been the subject of several learned statistical papers, including one by Kern.[10]

The object of Pass the Pigs® is to throw a pair of plastic pigs, evaluate the obtained score and then, depending on what happens, either throw them again, pass the pigs voluntarily to the next player or be forcibly required to do so. If both pigs land on their noses (which in 3939 throws carried out by 39 students, Freddie found to have a probability of 0.0016), this is known as a 'double snouter', and the lucky player gains 40 points. If both pigs land on their sides ('pig-out'), with their ears pointing towards each other (one with a dot facing up and one with a dot facing down), at an empirical probability of 0.105, the player forfeits all points for that turn and passes the pigs to the next player. The first player to reach 100 points wins. The game is not, as far as we know, played in any casinos, even Australian ones.

The moral of this story is that whether we are playing with a coin, two coins, dice, plastic pigs, animal bones, fire, love or life, we will generally do better at it if we understand the probabilities involved.

Probability distributions

Probability distributions include the binomial distribution and the normal probability distribution. The latter can be seen as a special case of the normal distribution that you were introduced to in Chapter 2 and allows us to calculate the probabilities of various events occurring. This provides the basis for inferences to be made from samples to populations with particular levels of certainty, which is the basis of inferential statistics. The characteristics of this distribution are known so well that this allows us to relate our sample values to underlying population values. This capability allows us to infer the probability that relationships such as differences or associations between our sample characteristics are true — as in true of their underlying populations, and not just of these samples. A central principle of the central limit theorem is that the larger the sample, the more likely its characteristics will reflect its underlying population characteristics. Sampling and how this relates to normal probability distributions will be covered in more detail in Chapter 5.

The binomial probability distribution

We can develop our description of probability distributions in the same way that we developed our description of probability theory — by beginning with a description of a type of probability distribution that plots a series of mutually exclusive binary possibilities. What then would be an example of a binary series of possibilities that we could plot on a binary probability distribution? If you enthusiastically answered 'coin tosses!', then you are well on your statistical way.

The binomial distribution can be seen as a discrete probability distribution of the number of successes in a series of yes/no events, each of which gives us a probability value of success. The binomial distribution can be approximated using the normal distribution, in that as the n gets large the binomial distribution starts to resemble a normal distribution. It should be noted, however, that this approximation is not good when probabilities are very low or very high, so (as with many things) it is more useful than perfect.

We can represent a binomial distribution as a histogram that gives us the frequencies of a series of binary events occurring (Fig 4.1). In this example we are interested in the probabilities of achieving 'heads' coin landing outcomes when two coins are thrown simultaneously (possibly because we have just bet on heads in a game of two-up). The distribution shown in Figure 4.1 gives us the three probabilities of coins coming up heads and this forms a normal distribution of probabilities. The probability of each of the events is plotted on the x axis, and the three outcomes of interest are plotted on the y axis. Defining a coin coming up heads as a 'success', Figure 4.1 shows the probability of 0, 1 and 2 successes for two trials (flips) for an event that has a probability of 0.50 of being a

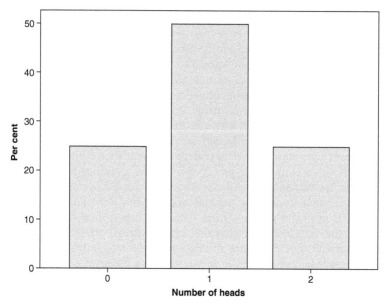

Fig 4.1   Binomial probability distribution histogram showing coin tossing results

success on each trial. This makes Figure 4.1 an example of a binomial distribution that allows us to answer such questions as: 'If two coins are thrown simultaneously, what is the probability of getting one or more heads?' Since the probability of getting exactly one head is 0.50 and the probability of getting exactly two heads is 0.25, the probability of getting one or more heads is 0.50 + 0.25 = 0.75.

The normal probability distribution

We can use the normal and other probability distributions to determine how well we can infer from a sample statistical finding to the true or population situation. If our research question involves comparing means, such as comparing the efficacy of two or more cancer treatments on a dimensional variable such as quality of life, we can use a probability distribution known as the sampling distribution of differences between means. This will tell us whether one or more treatments has performed significantly better than the others have. This difference can be expressed in terms of a p-value — the probability that the difference between means on an outcome measure for the treatments, such as quality of life, is statistically significant. The p-value is our chance (probability) of getting a result as large or larger than the one we have. Even more usefully, we can use confidence intervals to help us estimate the true population difference that underlies our sample.

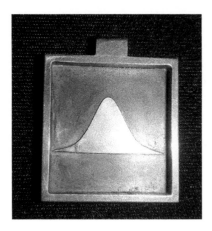

Fig 4.2 **The art of the normal probability distribution** (Ric Moodie/ Flickr)

Statistical significance is described in more detail in Chapter 6: basically if a result is statistically significant it means that there is a low probability (p) that we will be wrong if we state that our sample result is true of the population from which the sample was drawn, and not true just of our sample. Put simply, if we conducted a study 100 times, hypothetically we would expect a significant result less than 5 times if our significance level is 0.05 (see Chapter 6). It is important to note that we also have to calculate effect sizes to help assess the clinical significance of our results, as well as confidence intervals, so that we can put an interval around the estimate of the true population difference or whatever other relationship between samples interests us (see Chapter 6).

Subjective probability

There is an interesting area of probability known as subjective probability. This can be seen as a humanistic area of probability theory, in that it relates to people's belief in the chances of something happening. People's belief about the chances of something happening does not necessarily completely correspond with the actual chances of something happening. For example, there are people who fear flying far more than they fear driving, in the mistaken belief that flying is more dangerous than driving. The information evidence base clearly reveals, however, to anyone statistically literate enough to be interested in it, that driving is in fact far more dangerous than flying.

Another example of the difficulty that people often have with estimating probability involves the subjective comparison of the comparative mortalities associated with shark attacks and swimming pools. Swimming pool mortalities are far more common than shark attack mortalities, but if you asked a sample of your friends (or anyone else's) whether they should more actively avoid swimming pools or sharks, they may well base their response on something other than objective evidence. People's uncertainty about uncertainty may be caused by their being systematically distracted by potentially distorting features of information — such as that sharks are inherently (to most of us!) scarier than swimming pools. This phenomenon illustrates the potential health as well as health-science benefits of universal statistical literacy.

An alternative to subjective probability is the so-called frequentist view, which is based upon the observation of events (such as the frequency of coins coming up heads) over a long period of time (many coin tosses). If we throw enough coins, we would expect heads to come up half the time, although this may not happen if we are dealing with a small number of coin tosses.

An alternative to the frequentist view is the Bayesian view, originally developed in the UK by the Reverend Thomas Bayes (1702–61), a minister of religion and a mathematician. Very basically, Bayesian probability allows us a preliminary or prior estimate of a particular event happening — for example, that a coin might come up heads. This estimate can be based on long observation, a sober deduction that as there are two sides of a coin both may be equally likely to turn up, and so forth, or this can even be based on a wild hunch.

One of the criticisms levelled at Bayesian probability is the question of where the initial estimate comes from in the first place. What is known as Bayes's theorem allows us to revise our initial probability estimate on the basis of new information. If we are spending our evening in Nefarious Ned's Cactus Casino, for example, and notice that amid all the spitting and sawdust and swearing the coin really does seem to come up heads (when we are betting on heads) less frequently than our reasonable expectation of 50% of the time, we may legitimately grab our hats and depart. We may instead revise our initial 50% estimate based upon a fair coin, to one appropriate for a loaded one. This principle relates to the development of chess computers and other forms of artificial intelligence, where it has been found that giving a computer a capability of guessing and revising its guesses based on experience makes it far more successful ('intelligent') than just programming it to number-crunch.

Conclusion

This chapter has, possibly painlessly, introduced you to the underlying theory of probability, and also to probability distributions. Probability is a key concept in statistics that is used in inferential statistics to make inferences to populations on the basis of samples, with specified levels of certainty. In the next chapters the probability-related concepts covered in this one will be extended to an explanation of their role in the inferential statistics process, including hypothesis testing, sampling and the interpretation of statistical results.

Quick reference summary

• Probability theory was developed to meet particular needs, and these needs historically included those of gamblers to improve their chances of winning, or at least to better understand why they were losing.

• If we randomly throw a coin in the air, the probability of it coming down with either heads or tails facing up is exactly half, if we discount such wildly unlikely eventualities as the possibility it may land on its edge, or disappear into a previously unsuspected dimension, or be eaten by a homework-eating dog.

• Probability distributions include the binomial distribution and the normal probability distribution, and these allow us to calculate the probabilities of various events occurring.

• People's belief about the chances of something happening does not necessarily completely correspond with the actual chances of something happening.

• Statistically literate people are more likely than not quite so statistically literate people to base their beliefs about probability on objective evidence. This illustrates the potential health as well as health-science benefits of universal statistical literacy.

References

1. Maslow A. *Motivation and Personality*. New York: Harper; 1954.

2. Blackwood K. *Casino Gambling for Dummies*. New York: Wiley; 2006.

3. McKenzie DP, Onghena P, Hogenraad R, et al. Detecting patterns by one-sample runs tests: paradox, explanation and a new omnibus procedure. *Journal of Experimental Education*. 1999;67:167-179.

4. Ridley M. Why presidents have more sons. *New Scientist*. 1994;144:28-31.

5. Weaver W. *Lady Luck: the Theory of Probability*. New York: Dover; 1982.

6. Everitt BS. *Chance Rules: an Informal Guide to Probability, Risk, and Statistics*. 2nd ed. London: Springer; 2008.

7. Netuveli G, Pikhart H, Bobak M, et al. Generic quality of life predicts all-cause mortality in the short term: evidence from British Household Panel Survey. *Journal Epidemiologic Community Health.* 2012;66(10):962-966.

8. Fong TW, Campos MD, Brecht ML, et al. Problem and pathological gambling in a sample of casino patrons. *Journal Gambling Studies.* 2011;27(1):35-47.

9. Murrell PR. The statistics of Monopoly. *Chance.* 1999;12:36-40.

10. Kern J. Pig data and Bayesian influence on multinomial probabilities. *Journal of Statistics Education.* 2006;14(3).

Further reading

Altman DG, Machin D, Bryant TN, et al, eds. *Statistics with Confidence: Confidence Intervals and Statistical Guidelines.* 2nd ed. London: BMJ; 2000.

Haigh J. *Taking Chances: Winning with Probability.* 2nd ed. Oxford: Oxford University Press; 2003.

Howell D. *Statistical Methods for Psychology.* 7th ed. Belmont, CA: Duxbury Press; 2010.

Mazur J. *What's Luck Got to Do with It?: the History, Mathematics, and Psychology of the Gambler's Illusion.* Princeton, NJ: Princeton University Press; 2010.

CHAPTER 5

INFERENTIAL STATISTICS, SAMPLING AND HYPOTHESIS TESTING

All the business of war, and indeed all the business of life, is to endeavour to find out what you don't know by what you do.

ARTHUR WELLESLEY, DUKE OF WELLINGTON (1769–1852)

OBJECTIVES

After carefully reading this chapter you will understand the:

- basic nature of inferential statistics

- basic purpose of inferential statistics

- relationship between inferential statistics and probability theory

- difference between a null hypothesis and an alternative hypothesis

- difference between an appropriate inference and a rampant generalisation

- steps involved in using inferential statistics to help answer research and clinical questions.

Introduction

As mentioned in Chapter 3, statistics can conveniently be divided into (a) descriptive statistics, which can help us to make sense of our data by summarising and graphically displaying it, and (b) inferential statistics, which uses probability theory to help us extrapolate the characteristics of samples to populations. The inferential statistical process enables us to answer questions such as whether there are significant and also meaningful relationships (for example, differences or associations) in our measures of interest. If you liked descriptive statistics, or at least respected them for their descriptive power, then you might just *love* inferential statistics, for their potentially even greater inferential power.

Being able to make meaningful statements about populations — such as that one treatment will work better than another for relieving the symptoms of depressed people (our population), on the basis of trial data (our sample) — can be a highly valuable thing to do. An often unexpected positive side effect of the development of statistical literacy is that statistics, particularly inferential statistics, can be useful and even interesting, especially when applied to our own data.

People who lack statistical literacy tend to begin and end their statistical endeavours with descriptive statistics, whereas greater statistical adventures require a correct understanding and application of inferential statistics. Inferential statistics such as the Student t-test, Pearson correlation coefficient, Pearson chi-square, regression and Fisher's analysis of variance all allow us to generalise from a smaller set of data (sample) to a larger one (population), with a specified precision or with a measurable degree of confidence. You will learn more about these inferential statistical tests and others in later chapters, but you will be introduced to their common underlying principles here.

This chapter includes meaningful examples of inferential statistics in meaningful action; descriptions of how they relate to the probability theory that you were introduced to in Chapter 4; the nature of samples; the notion of degree of certainty that our sample-based population inferences are (a) accurate and (b) meaningful; and what errors to look out for in the application and interpretation of inferential statistics. This chapter will also describe some particular applications of inferential statistical procedure, including within a health-science research context.

A definition

Norman and Streiner pithily described inferential statistics as involving a process of inferring features of populations based on observations of samples.[1] Freund and Williams provided a more expansive definition of inferential statistics, or statistical inference, as involving reasoning from sample data to population parameters, which includes generalisations, predictions, estimates or decisions based on the sample.[2,3] A proviso could be added to the latter definition, to the effect that inferential statistical reasoning is best done in a logical and scientific manner, using accepted statistical methodology and principles. Otherwise, if an angry poodle or poodle-cross (our 'sample') chased us down the street one day, we might do more than be appropriately very descriptive indeed about that particular dog. If we then inferred that all poodles (our 'population') are best avoided on the basis of this one's behaviour (our 'sample'), we are not displaying statistical literacy and are perhaps unready for a job as a statistician (or mobile dog washer).

Sampling

Inferential statistics allow us to make inferences from samples to their underlying populations, so it is important to know something about the nature of samples and what distinguishes a good one from a not-quite-so-good one, before being introduced to particular inferential statistics.

What do you think would make a good sample? To put this question another way, what characteristics would a sample need for you to feel comfortable in making generalisations about your population of interest based on it? A sample needs to be representative of our population for us to be comfortable that our sample results are an accurate reflection of the characteristics of our entire population. If every member of a population has an equal chance of ending up in our sample, we probably have a representative sample. If there is a reason why some members of a population have a greater chance of being included in our sample than others, whether we know about this reason or not, our sample is probably distorted and is not fully representative of our population.

Characteristics of good samples

There are some important characteristics of an appropriately selected research sample that you should incorporate in your own research, and look for in other people's research. Samples will need to display these characteristics in order to be representative enough of their underlying populations to enable researchers to confidently make inferences about the populations based on their sample results. Firstly, the larger a sample is, the more likely it is to provide an accurate reflection of its underlying population or, in slightly less technical terms, the bigger the better (generally). There is a statistical technique known as power analysis that can be used to calculate appropriate sample sizes for our particular research needs. A detailed description of this is outside of the scope of this introduction to sampling, but the active ingredient of this technique is the common principle underlying appropriate sampling — the bigger the better.

Determining an optimal sample size relates to the everyday and non-technical concept of familiarity — we tend to trust people and situations that we know well better than we trust people and situations that we do not know well, because we are more familiar with their behaviour and nature. To relate familiarity to sampling, the more observations of a behaviour that we have, the more familiar we are with it, and the more comfortable we are likely to be in inferring characteristics from these observations (our sample data: *some* behaviours of this person) to our general opinion of this person (our population: *all* behaviours of this person). The better we know something, the more likely we are to trust it, whether the something we are trusting is sample data or any other observations, and therefore the more observations of a population that we have (the larger our sample), the more likely it is to be representative of the population from which it was drawn.

Random selection

A common way of ensuring that there is no systematic bias in our sample is by selecting on the basis of chance, via the *random sampling* of participants. There are commonly used methods for achieving the random selection of members of a population, such as random number generation, and these are designed to ensure that research participants are selected in a manner that gives every member of the population an equal chance of being selected. A form of random sampling that can be very useful, particularly in situations where it is difficult to obtain suitably large sample numbers, is *stratified random sampling*. This process can involve the division of the population of interest into segments (strata) and sampling within the strata of interest. Researchers can ensure that their sample contains the same proportion of people from each of the identified strata as are in the entire population, which improves the sample's representativeness.

Characteristics of not-so-good samples

A sample is more likely to be an accurate reflection of an underlying population when it is large, but just being large does not guarantee a sample's representativeness. It is possible to select a large sample from a population that is unrepresentative, especially when there is a systematic bias at play.

Samples will not be fully representative of their populations if they are distorted by some form of systematic selection bias. A common way of systematically distorting the representativeness of a sample is using *convenience samples*. A convenience sample is, perhaps unsurprisingly, one that is obtained on the basis of convenience, rather than on the basis of ensuring that every member of the population of interest has an equal chance of being selected in the sample.

A common real-research example of a convenience sample is where the researcher tests people who just happen to be conveniently physically proximate, rather like a giant spider with a grant waiting for unsuspecting flies to enter its research web. Although often convenient for a busy researcher, this approach to sampling risks a systematic biasing of the sample results — for example, the people walking past a researcher's door might be more likely to be from a certain sector of the community than from another sector. Students, young people and researchers are likely to be over-represented in this type of convenience sample. A convenience sample may therefore not be truly representative of the entire population to which the researcher wants to generalise the research findings.

It is likely that convenient sample selection is universally influencing the results of health-science research, in that first-year health-science students are greatly over-represented in research samples. Dan Jones made the point in his 2010 *Science* article, for example, that most psychology research is conducted on *WEIRDos* — people from **W**estern, **e**ducated, **i**ndustrialised, **r**ich and **d**emocratic cultures, and are therefore not necessarily fully representative of the population (everybody everywhere) to which researchers are usually interested in generalising their results.[4] It could further be mentioned that health-science research participants are probably unrepresentatively young and possibly unrepresentatively intelligent. This important observation does not mean that health-science research should be globally dismissed, but that we should always carefully evaluate the context of research results, whether these are ours or those of other people.

Sample selection bias: a historical example

A striking real-life, historical general example of the potentially profound effects of sample selection bias involves political science rather than health science, but it universally demonstrates how statistics can go very wrong if they are not used very carefully. In 1948 a relatively new statistical science application — the opinion poll — 'scientifically proved' that Republican candidate Thomas E Dewey would easily defeat Harry S Truman in the United States presidential election. Dewey knew enough about inferential statistics to make them dangerous — he unquestionably believed in them. Dewey's statistical belief was so strong that on the strength of what statistics seemed to be telling him he tentatively booked a 5000-person reception centre to celebrate his impending victory. Fortunately, he did not pay a deposit.

All of the 1948 major political pollsters including Gallup and Roper predicted a Dewey win in the 1948 election.[4] Worse still, on the morning of 3 November 1948, the *Chicago Daily Tribune* ran the headline 'DEWEY DEFEATS TRUMAN'. According to reality, however, rather than misused statistics, Harry S Truman had in fact won the election. This unfortunate fact so embarrassed the senior staff of the *Chicago Daily Tribune* that they rushed out onto the streets to physically retrieve copies of their paper with its infamously wrong headline. What Thomas E Dewey and the pollsters

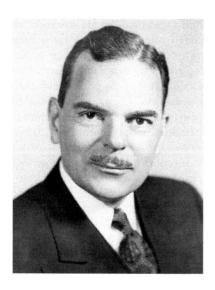

Fig 5.1   Thomas E Dewey, a key
player in a famous historical
example of sample selection bias
in an opinion poll

forgot to infer from their inferential statistics was that, in order to be accurate, samples have to be representative of the populations from which they are taken, even when the sample is enormous.

Can you think of a form of systematic sample bias that may have influenced the results of the 1948 USA presidential election opinion polls? Was there something important that the opinion pollsters did not take account of in their sampling? In 1948 there was a group of people who were less likely to respond if the telephone was used to ask who they intended to vote for. This group consisted of people who did not have a phone, and many of them did not have one because they were too poor to be able to afford one. In 1948 (and possibly now) poor people in the USA were more likely to vote Democrat than Republican, which meant that not every member of the population (all USA voters) had an equal chance of being included in the samples (telephone opinion polls). This statistical malpractice led to the failure of opinion polls to predict that Dewey would be beaten by Truman in what almost everyone at the time thought was an astonishingly strange result. This statistical story is a classic illustration of how it is possible to be information rich but wisdom poor, and of the importance of using statistics wisely.

Sample selection bias: a health-science example

A study conducted at the Department of Obstetrics and Gynecology, University of Utah School of Medicine, explored whether there might be a systematic bias affecting the results of genetic specimen tests that could affect their generalisation.[5] The researchers were interested in whether women who agreed to the future use of their maternal and fetal DNA samples, including testing for research purposes, might not be fully representative of all women.

The potential systematic sample bias in genetic testing research involved 5003 of 5188 women enrolled in a multicentre observational study that was originally designed to test for a particular genetic mutation (factor V Leiden). Approximately 80% of the research participants agreed to having their genetic samples stored (and used for research), and it was found that black, Hispanic and tobacco-using women were under-represented in this group. The researchers concluded that the study sample of women agreeing to the storage and research use of their genetic samples was not fully representative of the population to which genetic researchers are usually interested in generalising — that is, all women. Population inferences made on the basis of this sample may not, therefore, have been completely accurate.

Hypothesis testing

The null hypothesis

It is possible to apply statistics to the testing of our research question in much the same way that some people use private investigators and palm readers — merely to confirm our suspicions. In order to reduce the likelihood of such statistical misdemeanours, we therefore generally commence our statistical testing by generating a *null hypothesis*. This is the stated assumption that there is no significant relationship between our variables of interest, such as differences or associations. This is the statistical equivalent of the legal assumption that defendants are presumed innocent until the weight of evidence against them establishes their guilt, beyond reasonable doubt. In statistics, the null hypothesis remains true (or rather, is not rejected) until there is sufficient evidence that there is a significant statistical finding, such as a genuine difference between experimental conditions, or a genuine association between variables.

We test the results of our statistical analyses against a null hypothesis because it is good scientific practice (and also good general practice) to be objective and not to be influenced by our expectations, and therefore to undertake our statistical analyses with an open mind. Scientific open-mindedness involves a calm and honest appraisal of the available evidence, and then accepting or rejecting it according to objective and previously defined criteria. Beginning our statistical testing procedure with the generation of a null hypothesis means that the onus is on us, the researchers, to objectively demonstrate that a genuine statistical finding has been achieved. This procedure resembles the practice in many legal systems, where the onus is on the prosecution to objectively demonstrate a genuine legal finding.

A health-science example

A health-science example of the generation of a null hypothesis could commence with our research interest in the relationship between day of the week and likelihood of suffering a heart attack. There are various ways that we could investigate this research question, including testing whether there is a significant association between day of the week and likelihood of suffering a heart attack, or testing whether there is a significant difference between heart attack incidence on the different days of the week. Our null hypothesis in the first research situation will state that there is no association between day of the week and the likelihood of heart attack. Our null hypothesis in the second research situation will state that there is no difference between the number of heart attacks occurring on different days of the week.

The alternative hypothesis

Once we have a research question and a null hypothesis, we need a formal expression of the possibility that there is indeed a significant relationship contained within our variables of interest, such as a real association between scores on our variables of interest, or a real difference in scores on our dependent variable between conditions of our independent variable. We can express this alternative possibility by generating an alternative, or experimental, hypothesis. Our alternative hypothesis can be seen as the stated possibility that what we think might be true of our results is indeed true, beyond reasonable doubt.

We need an a priori (before the event, i.e. before the statistical analysis) logical reason for generating an alternative hypothesis, which can be based on our comprehensive reading about our topic of interest, or on our clinical observations, or on our logical expectations based on compelling theoretical grounds, or on all of the above.

A health-science example

We might expect that heart attack likelihood is related to day of the week, which means that we can appropriately generate a specific alternative (to the null) hypothesis that states that heart attack likelihood is associated with day of the week. We can then test this hypothesis by using an appropriate inferential statistical test (described in a later chapter). In the case of an expected difference in heart attack incidence between days of the week, our alternative hypothesis could be that there will be a significant difference in our dependent variable — heart attack incidence — between the conditions (days of the week) of our independent variable.

Directional and non-directional hypotheses

The second alternative hypothesis described above is *non-directional*, because it does not nominate an expected direction of difference. We could also generate a directional alternative hypothesis, which nominates an expected direction of difference, such as that heart attack likelihood will be higher on a particular day or days of the week than it will be on other days. If we have generated a directional alternative hypothesis, then technically it is appropriate for us to use a *one-tailed test* of the significance of our difference result. If we have a non-directional hypothesis, then technically it is appropriate for us to use a *two-tailed test* (two directions) of the significance of our difference result. In practice, however, we usually generate a directional hypothesis, but still use a two-tailed (non-directional) test of statistical significance because it is more conservative — that is, less likely to lead to an erroneous result.

Directional hypotheses are rarely used in contemporary statistical research (or anywhere else for that matter) because of their lack of conservatism. We are more likely to reject our null hypothesis — the presumption of statistical innocence — when we use one-tailed tests (types of hypothesis-testing errors will be described in later sections). This is why many good statistical judges, such as research journal editors, can be suspicious of the use of one-tailed statistical tests. It is possible to undertake research and to statistically analyse research findings without stating any research hypotheses, but such research needs to be focused by some objective criterion that reduces the potentially infinite and infinitely meaningless range of associated possible research outcomes. Research that examines the results of a great many variables without stating what results are logically expected is often disparagingly described as a shot-gun approach, or a fishing expedition, or (far more respectfully) data mining.

Hypothesis testing epilogue

We can use inferential statistics either to reject or to fail to reject our null hypothesis, and therefore indirectly support our alternative hypothesis. We can do this by applying an appropriate test of significance to the results of an appropriate statistical test. Which statistical test and associated significance test is appropriate for us to use will depend on the nature of our research question, and on the nature of our chosen research design. No matter which significance test we use to test our null hypothesis, we need to follow appropriate general inferential statistical significance testing conventions, which will be described below.

Inferential statistical testing procedure

You may have initially considered inferential statistics to have a very narrow application, and perhaps to be only an ongoing source of fascination and delight to statisticians, and other non-normally distributed life forms. Inferential statistics, however, are actually highly useful in the real, or at least realistic, world that surrounds and sometimes informs us, including the health-science world. Some examples of inferential statistics in general and health-science specific action will now be provided.

A general example

A good everyday (or at least every thousand or so days) example of both descriptive and inferential statistics in action — together — can readily be found in the media coverage of elections. State-of-the-science super-computers (that traditionally run out of steam halfway through the tele-cast) are typically employed to predict winners, based on a slowly increasing vote count. This constitutes an increasingly large sample of the eventual population of total votes cast.

You might remember from the last election coverage you watched on the TV or listened to on the radio (or you might notice the next time you tune in to such a coverage) that the highly statistically literate experts who are often employed to appear on these election coverages typically dazzle us with impressively presented descriptive data. These descriptive data presentations typically include pie charts or bar graphs that indicate, colourfully, that our current government is doomed because it is cur-rently trailing by 88% to 12% of the current vote. The election statistical experts often then inform us sagely (and appropriately) that we should soberly totally disregard these early results (if we are able to), because they are based on a meaninglessly tiny sample. These statistical experts then usually confess that we need a much larger sample size before we can appropriately infer a likely population result: that is, suggest who will win the election.

With our new statistical savvy we can now ask why they bothered to show us inferentially statistically meaningless information in the first place. We can also ask just how long we will need to wait for an inferential, statistically meaningful result based on the increasing vote sample size — a good election outcome guess.

A health-science example

We can use a new and interesting health-science research example to illustrate the entire inferential statistical sequence from hypothesis genera-tion and testing to significance testing.

Background

In 1973 David Rosenhan published a research paper in the well-respected journal *Science* that was thought-provokingly entitled 'On being sane in insane places'.[6] Rosenhan's study investigated the validity of psychiatric diagnoses in two ways. The first phase of the study consisted of experi-mental confederates achieving admission to 12 psychiatric institutions around the USA by faking common symptoms of mental illnesses, such as auditory hallucinations. The 12 'pseudopatients' then displayed per-fectly normal behaviour once they were institutionalised, but none of their psychiatric diagnoses were rescinded. The second phase of this study was precipitated when one of the psychiatric institutions that was offended by Rosenhan's results challenged him to send them more 'pseudopatients', so that they would have an opportunity to rescind inaccurate ongoing diagnoses. The hospital subsequently rescinded the initial diagnoses of 41 of their 193 new patients, therefore identifying 41 'pseudopatients', based on their apparent postadmission 'normal' behaviour. In fact, Rosenhan had sent the hospital zero 'pseudopatients'.

Follow-ups to Rosenhan's experiment have included a study conducted by Marti Loring and Brian Powell in 1988.[7] This study included an inferential statistical exploration of whether there is an ongoing systematic bias in psychiatric diagnosis, specifically resulting in such diagnoses being affected by the gender and race characteristics of potential psychiatric patients. This research was undertaken in the context of the researchers' interest in whether the introduction of the standardised tool for diagnosing mental illness — the Diagnostic and Statistical Manual (DSM)[8] — had resulted in increased objectivity of psychiatric diagnoses since David Rosenhan's 1973 experiment.

The research sequence

Loring and Powell's research began with a research question: whether the psychiatric diagnoses of a range of common psychiatric disorders were influenced by demographic factors such as people's gender and race. The researchers then devised a research program and statistical analysis that was designed to allow this research question to be answered objectively. A sample of 290 psychiatrists were recruited to the experiment and each was then asked to diagnose 'cases' that were variously described as relating to a white male, a white female, a black male, a black female and to others with gender and race undisclosed. In order to give an objective answer to the research question of whether there is an association between likelihood of psychiatric diagnosis and (a) gender or (b) race, specific null hypotheses needed to be generated, which can be tested by subsequent inferential statistical tests and associated significance testing:

Null hypothesis 1 (H0 1). There is no association between a person's gender and the likelihood of being given a psychiatric diagnosis.

Null hypothesis 2 (H0 2). There is no association between a person's race and the likelihood of being given a psychiatric diagnosis.

Two associated alternative (experimental) hypotheses now needed to be generated:

Alternative hypothesis 1 (H1): There is an association between a person's gender and the likelihood of being given a psychiatric diagnosis,

Alternative hypothesis 2 (H2): There is an association between a person's race and the likelihood of being given a psychiatric diagnosis.

The statistical tests that were applied in this study included the correlation inferential statistic that calculates the degree of association between variables, which will be described fully in Chapter 8. The results of this correlation analysis showed that (a) there was a significant positive association between gender and likelihood of being given a psychiatric diagnosis (females were more likely to be diagnosed), and (b) there was a significant positive association between race and likelihood of being given a psychiatric diagnosis (blacks were more likely to be diagnosed). These correlations were significant at the 0.05 level, which meant that there was less than a 5% chance that this sample result (of 290 psychiatrists) was not also true of the underlying population (all psychiatrists). The null hypotheses — there is no association between (1) gender and psychiatric diagnosis likelihood or (2) race and psychiatric diagnosis likelihood — can therefore be rejected. This provides (indirect) support for the two alternative hypotheses — there *is* an association between (1) gender and psychiatric diagnosis likelihood or (2) race and psychiatric diagnosis likelihood. It was concluded on the basis of the results of this research that, despite the objective diagnostic criteria offered by the DSM, there was a subjective component of psychiatric diagnoses.

It should be noted that the working definition of a population to which we are making our inferential statistical generalisations, on the basis of our sample results, is not always as clear cut as it may seem, even to experienced researchers. For example, is the population in the above research example *all psychiatrists, everywhere, over all times*, or just *American psychiatrists in 1973*? With a more detailed knowledge of the manner in which the above sample was obtained, it may be possible to generate further reductions in the scope of the population to which the sample results relate. A key point that arises here is that being statistically literate often means knowing what questions to ask.

Conclusion

Now that you know something about the nature of inferential statistics and the research sequence within which they are normally conducted, the next step is for you to learn something useful about significance testing and experimental design, before learning something useful about some particular commonly used inferential statistical tests. Measures of difference will be covered in Chapters 7 and 8, and measures of association will be covered in Chapters 9 and 10.

Quick reference summary

- Inferential statistics allows us to make inferences from samples to their underlying populations.

- A sample needs to be representative of its population for us to be comfortable that our sample results are an accurate reflection of the characteristics of our population.

- Samples will not be fully representative of their populations if they are distorted by some form of systematic selection bias.

- To be objective and to avoid being influenced by our expectations, we test the results of our statistical analyses against a null hypothesis.

References

1. Norman GR, Streiner DL. *PDQ Statistics.* 3rd ed. Hamilton, Ontario: BC Decker; 2003.

2. Freund JF, Williams FJ. *Dictionary/Outline of Basic Statistics.* New York: Dover; 1991 [Originally published in 1966 by McGraw-Hill, New York.]

3. Gallup G. *The Gallup Poll; Public Opinion, 1935–1971.* New York: Random House; 1972.

4. Jones D. A WEIRD view of human nature skews psychologists' studies. *Science.* 2010;328(5986):1627.

5. Aagaard-Tillery K, Sibai B, Spong CY, et al. Sample bias among women with retained DNA samples for future genetic studies. *Obstetric Gynecology.* 2006;108(5):1115-1120.

6. Rosenhan DL. On being sane in insane places. *Science.* 1973;179(4070):250-258.

7. Loring M, Powell B. Gender, race, and DSM-III: a study of the objectivity of psychiatric diagnostic behavior. *Journal of Health and Social Behaviour.* 1988;29(1):1-22.

8. *The Diagnostic and Statistical Manual of Mental Disorders.* 3rd ed. Washington DC: American Psychiatric Association; 1980.

CHAPTER 6

SIGNIFICANCE TESTING, BEYOND SIGNIFICANCE TESTING, AND EXPERIMENTAL DESIGN

To generalize is to be an idiot.

WILLIAM BLAKE (1757–1827)

OBJECTIVES

After carefully reading this chapter you will:

- know the significance of statistical significance

- be confident about the meaning and application of confidence intervals

- be clear on the difference between a significant result and a meaningful result

- have some familiarity with some major types of experimental design

- recognise that life itself can be a (vital) experiment.

Introduction

We can use significance testing to help us to appropriately infer from the characteristics of samples to the characteristics of populations. This process makes use of probability theory, which was covered in Chapter 4, to statistically test our hypotheses, which were described in Chapter 5. It is important to know that there is more to the inferential statistical story than statistical significance and that, just because a result is statistically significant, it does not have to mean that the result is also clinically meaningful. This chapter will therefore cover effect sizes and confidence intervals. You will also be introduced to the major types of experimental design.

Significance testing

We can use significance testing to test our hypotheses in relation to the characteristics of our variables of interest, such as associations or differences. If our statistical test leads to a statistically significant result, such as a significantly high level of association or difference between our variables of interest, we can infer that our sample result is not just true of our sample but also of our populations of interest. The calculation of statistical significance makes use of probability theory, which was introduced in Chapter 4, and uses random sampling distributions to help us answer questions such as whether our two sample means are likely to come from the same population (in which case the null hypothesis *cannot* be rejected) or from different populations (in which case the null hypothesis *can* be rejected).

We use significance testing in inferential statistics because in research we are often interested in whether our results can be generalised. If, for example, we find that the incidence of heart attacks is greater on one day of the week than it is on another day, this finding is only of value if this difference can be generalised from our sample to a population — for example, all potential heart attack sufferers. Sample results — such as a finding that that one group of people scored higher or lower on a particular dependent variable than did another group, or that their scores on two variables of interest are associated — do not provide us with useful information in themselves. We also need to know whether these differences or associations are due to the idiosyncratic or distorted nature of our sample, or whether they are in fact true in that they can be generalised to our samples' underlying populations.

Some health-science examples

To conclude the heart-attack incidence example to which you were introduced in Chapter 5, a group of researchers in Austria found that there is a significant difference between days of the week in the likelihood of heart attack occurring. Heart-attack incidence is higher on Mondays than it is on other days. The interpretation of this inferential statistical result is not clear cut, but the researchers suggested that that there may be a stress-inducing event that tends to systematically occur on Mondays![1]

There is also a phenomenon known as the 'weekend effect'. People who are admitted to hospital at weekends with serious conditions such as heart attacks are less likely to recover than people who are admitted to hospital on weekdays with the same conditions. A 2010 Australian study of 17,809 acute myocardial infarction hospital admissions showed that patients who were admitted over a weekend were highly significantly less likely to recover than were patients who were admitted on a weekday.[2] The reason for this result is also unclear, but may relate to decreased access to medical procedures at weekends.

Levels of significance

There is a convention in inferential statistics that there generally needs to be less than a 5% chance that we falsely reject our null hypothesis before we can reject it. Another way of saying this is that there needs to be less than 1 chance in 20 of falsely rejecting our null hypothesis or thinking there is a result when there is not (because it is actually due to chance). The criterion of 5%, or 1 in 20, is arbitrary, but this is widely enough accepted to be considered meaningful. Before carrying out hypothesis tests, it is necessary for us to specify an *alpha level* — a probability level or a standard beneath which our obtained probability level will be deemed to be statistically significant. If we are being particularly conservative (or confident!) in our hypothesis testing, we can nominate an alpha level of 0.01 (less than a 1%, or 1 in 100, chance that our null hypothesis will actually be true before we reject it) or even 0.001 (less than a 0.1%, or 1 in 1000 chance that our null hypothesis will actually be true before we reject it).

If our probability of obtaining a test result as large as or larger than the one we obtained (if the null hypothesis is in fact true) is less than 0.05, this result will be reported as '$p < 0.05$'. Such a happy result will therefore be deemed to be statistically significant. If our probability of obtaining a test result as large or larger than the one we obtained (if the null hypothesis is true) is less than 0.01, this result will be reported as $p < 0.01$ and is more statistically significant. If our probability of obtaining a result as large or larger than the one we obtained is less than 0.001, this result will be reported as $p < 0.001$, and we could perhaps throw a party or apply for a research grant to celebrate. If we are statistically literate, however, we might not do this unless we have a *meaningful* result, as well as a *statistically significant* one, and the difference is explained and illustrated in the following sections.

Significance testing error types

There are two basic types of error that we can make in statistical significance testing. The first is rejecting our null hypothesis when it is in fact true. This potential error is known as a *type 1 error*, which is a 'false alarm' or 'false positive', and can be described as an error of *optimism* — for example, when a researcher wrongly rejects the assumption that the research result is actually non-significant. This type of error is conceptually equivalent to a prosecutor successfully obtaining a guilty verdict against a person who is actually innocent of their alleged crime.

The second error that we can make in our significance testing is failing to reject the null hypothesis when it should be rejected. This error is known as a *type 2 error*, which is a 'false negative', and can be described as an error of *pessimism* — for example, when a researcher wrongly fails to reject the assumption that the research result is non-significant.

In statistical hypothesis testing, there is a trade-off between the chances of making a type 1 error and the chances of making a type 2 error. If the alpha is set too low (to minimise the chances of making a type 1 error), we will risk missing real population relationships in our sample data, such as differences and associations between groups of scores. In this case we are being too conservative. If the alpha is set too high (to minimise the chances of making a type 2 error), we will risk claiming that there is something significant in our data when in fact there is not. In this case we are being too liberal.

A general example of this trade-off principle is the case of the boy (or girl) who cried wolf. If you aren't old enough to remember Aesop (620– 564 BC) or his fables, the child who cried wolf was a young shepherd who thought it fun to scare his villagers by shouting 'Wolf!' when there *wasn't* one, and who eventually learned a powerfully painful lesson when he cried 'Wolf!' when there *was* one. This boy achieved fame (or notoriety) for making a type 1 significance testing error — that is, reporting a significant finding (a wolf) when in fact there was nothing objectively significant in his data (sensory experience). If the boy who cried wolf had subsequently traded some of his sensory optimism for some sensory conservatism, he may have achieved a far greater level of scientific credibility.

Beyond statistical significance

Knowing whether or not our inferential statistical results are statistically significant is not the end of our inferential statistical story. We also need to know whether our results are meaningful, which in the area of health-science research often means *clinically meaningful*. There is an increasing tendency in the reporting of inferential statistical results for *effect size* and *confidence intervals* to be reported, in addition to measures of statistical significance. This is a welcome indication that perhaps the research world, and possibly the entire world, is becoming more statistically literate. Effect sizes (with a research example of their importance) and confidence intervals (and their underlying principles) are briefly outlined in the following sections. They will be described in more detail in Chapters 7 and 9, in the context of examples of two inferential statistical tests to which they are commonly applied.

Effect size

A potential problem with interpreting significance test results is that with a large enough sample size even a trivial result can be statistically significant, such as a very small difference or association between sets of scores. We therefore need measures of how meaningful our statistical results are, as well as measures of whether or not they are statistically significant.

A good way of discovering whether our results are meaningful as well as statistically significant is to calculate a measure of effect size, and indeed many journals now insist on such measures being reported in addition to significance levels. Jacob Cohen (1923–98) was a distinguished psychologist who gave the world many important and useful statistical techniques, and one of these was Cohen's d measure of effect size. This measure can be used in various ways, including taking variance into account when calculating an effect size for the differences between group means. Other measures of effect size, such as the eta-squared and the r-squared, which are used to calculate effect size within the context of particular inferential statistical tests, will be described in Chapters 7 and 9. What is common to all of these measures of effect size is that they help to tell us how meaningful our results are, as well as how statistically significant.

A health-science example
of the importance of effect size

In Chapter 1 you were briefly introduced to a meta-analysis-based study by Kirsch and colleagues of the efficacy of antidepressants,[3] as an interesting and elucidating example of clinically relevant research and research statistics. This study is also a good example of the importance of effect size in health-science research and research-related clinical practice. You might remember that Kirsch found on the basis of his statistical analysis of many studies of the efficacy of antidepressants, including unpublished studies, that antidepressants are not useful in the treatment of mild and moderate depression, and that they are only useful in the treatment of severe depression.

As you might have guessed, Kirsch's research caused quite a stir in depression research and clinical practice circles. As you might also have guessed, this research led to a substantial number of responses, including some particularly statistically well-reasoned ones. Möller made the point that the interpretation of Kirsch's results depends on aspects of effect-size reporting that are actually somewhat mysterious.[4] Such mysteries could be said to include the arbitrary conventions for designating what constitutes a clinically meaningful effect size, such as a Cohen's d measure. If one were to apply a less rigorous interpretation of what constitutes a meaningful Cohen's d effect size than was suggested by Cohen, it could be argued that antidepressants are indeed (perhaps marginally) useful for treating mild and moderate depression. That so much can hang on such statistical niceties as these demonstrates the vital importance of applying statistics, and their underlying principles, very carefully indeed.

Confidence intervals

A potential problem with interpreting inferential statistical significance test results is that understanding a result only in terms of whether or not it is statistically significant can be limiting and even misleading. Confidence intervals are a way of describing experimental results that can give us more useful information than hypothesis testing alone can. The basic nature of statistical hypothesis testing is that it is binary — a null hypothesis is either retained or rejected. Similarly, in statistical significance testing the results tends to be seen only as being either significant or not significant. Confidence intervals allow us to make more expansive interpretations of our results, and this is one reason why they are (appropriately) becoming increasingly commonly calculated and reported.

An important advantage of calculating and reporting confidence intervals, as well as significance test results, is that they allow us to go beyond statements such as that two group means are significantly different from each other. With a 95% confidence of this being true (of the underlying population) or, strictly speaking, if we ran an unlimited number of studies and calculated confidence intervals for each, 95% of them would actually contain the true or actual population value. Calculating confidence intervals in addition to calculating statistical significance allows us to ask questions that will be potentially more informative than those we can ask if we calculate statistical significance alone — for example: what is the range of differences between two group sample means that we are 95% confident are true, as in true of their underlying populations? In the day-of-the-week heart attack incidence example, we can calculate confidence intervals to tell us more than that there is a significant difference between different day-of-the-week sample means. Confidence intervals could be used to tell us the likely range of difference between heart attacks on a Monday and heart attacks on other days.

Confidence intervals can also be used to place a range of likely scores around a particular sample score, at a designated level of confidence. In intelligence testing, for example, the test result could be seen as a sample of an underlying population of all possible sample results for the person taking the test. An individual's test results are potentially affected by factors such as their current levels of fatigue and motivation, and it is not appropriate to state with certainty that an individual has a particular intelligence test score or, worse still, a particular intelligence. Instead of stating that an individual has for example an IQ of 112, it is better to state, on the basis of the calculation of a confidence interval, that we are (for example) 95% confident that their true (population) IQ score lies within a particular range, such as from 107 to 117. In choosing a confidence level (for example, 95% or 99%) for confidence intervals, we should remember that there is a trade-off between level of confidence and width of the confidence interval. Increasing the confidence interval will also increase the width of the confidence interval, so in the case of the intelligence test example if we wanted to be 99% rather than 95% confident of the range of true scores, the range would increase. This increase could be, for example, from being 95% confident that the true test score is between 112 and 117, to being 99% confident that the true score is between 104 and 120. Health-science examples of confidence intervals calculated in the context of particular statistics are given in Chapters 7 and 9.

Types of experimental design

Research can usefully be divided into fully experimental, quasi-experimental, observational and correlational. The nature of experimental design will depend on a range of interrelated factors, including the research question and the data to which it leads. The nature of the experimental design will also determine which statistical procedures we need to select and apply (see Chapters 7–12). In this section some major types of experimental design are covered briefly; for more detail on this topic, see Maxwell and Delaney.[5]

Fully experimental designs

The basic aim of experimental research is to find out something that we do not currently know; we experiment to help us find new information by systematically adding conditions to test against other conditions. Many of us conduct experiments without necessarily even knowing that we are doing so, such as when we seek to discover the best way to drive home by systematically testing route A against route B, or to discover the best or cheapest restaurant in our neighbourhood by systematically comparing restaurant A with restaurants B and C.

In a fully experimental research design, the researcher manipulates a variable or variables (the independent variable[s]) and this causes changes to another variable or variables (the dependent variable[s]). The dependent variable is so named because its values are dependent on those of the independent variable, and this can be seen as a measure of the phenomenon that interests us. It is important that any relationship observed between independent variables is due to differences between independent variables, and not to extraneous factors such as individual differences between people in different experimental conditions, fatigue or a practice effect. In fully experimental designs we therefore need to control to the best of our ability for the possible influence of such extraneous (uncontrolled) variables.

Some common types of extraneous or potentially extraneous variables are:

1. environment-related — for example, the potential effects on the dependent variable(s) of testing at different times of day or in different physical situations

2. participant-related — for example, the potential effects on the dependent variable(s) of participants' age, gender, socioeconomic status, fatigue and increasing familiarity with a test.

The possible uncontrolled effects of extraneous variables can be reduced if researchers hold all conditions associated with their experiments as constant as possible, apart from those that are deliberately being manipulated. This control of conditions can be assisted by using identical instructions, testing all participants at the same time of day and testing only people of the same age or with other potentially influential characteristics. Other ways of reducing the effects of extraneous variables include matching experimental participants on potentially relevant characteristics and randomly assigning them to experimental conditions, so that potentially extraneous influences will be distributed evenly between experimental groups.

Examples of experimental designs are given in later chapters that cover particular inferential statistical techniques: for t-tests in Chapter 7 and for analysis of variance (ANOVA) see Chapter 8. For a broad theoretical discussion of the nature of the prevailing experimental paradigm that is operating within a particular area of health-science research, see Valsiner.[6] This author suggests that there is a need to expand and evolve the prevailing experimental paradigm in at least one area of health-science research so as to produce a universal science, that is context-sensitive and culture-inclusive.

Quasi-experimental designs

This type of research is similar to fully experimental research, except that in quasi-experimental research the researcher has less control over the experimental design. This may mean, for example, that the researcher does not control the allocation of participants to experimental conditions nor use random selection. In quasi-experimental designs, there is therefore generally a weaker causal relationship between treatment conditions and outcomes. Despite this, the practicalities of research sometimes result in situations where fully experimental designs are not appropriate and quasi-experimental designs are adopted.

An interesting example of a quasi-experimental research brings together a broad approach to health and science. Some researchers in New Jersey investigated the clinical efficacy of reiki therapy (healing hands) for relieving pain and anxiety in women with abdominal hysterectomies.[7] Two small samples of women were tested after abdominal hysterectomy. The experimental group received traditional nursing care plus reiki (three 30-minute sessions), and the control group received traditional nursing care. The results of this study indicated statistically significant benefits of the reiki treatment addition, with the reiki-treated group reporting less pain, anxiety and requesting fewer analgesics than the control group. The design of this research study was quasi-experimental rather than experimental, because participants in it were not randomly assigned to the research conditions.

Observational designs

There are research situations where it is not possible to manipulate experimental conditions in order to demonstrate a clear causal relationship between conditions, such as treatment versus no treatment, and outcomes. It may be the case, for example, that it is unethical to withhold a treatment that may be beneficial from one group of people; or it may not be possible to manipulate conditions because they are beyond the researcher's control — for example, naturally occurring conditions/outcomes such as the psychological effects of exposure to a natural disaster. In situations such as these, researchers do not manipulate experimental conditions and directly relate outcomes to differences between conditions, but instead observe and describe phenomena rather than induce them.

An example of an observational design is offered by research conducted in France into factors associated with non-treatment compliance in women with breast cancer.[8] Medical records of 926 women across 99 hospitals were examined, and the women were divided on this basis into categories of 'compliant', 'justifiable' and 'not compliant'. Non-compliance factors were identified and included medical factors (such as severity of the illness) and organisational factors (such as the region of healthcare). This study was observational rather than experimental because the research conditions were not manipulated, but observed, via an analysis of medical records. In this situation it would obviously not have been ethical to have systematically manipulated research conditions.

Correlational designs

In correlational designs there is no attempt to establish a causal relationship between experimental conditions and outcomes. Correlations and correlational design will be fully covered in Chapter 9, but can be summarily described here as providing measures of association between variables. The following brief example is from the author's current research into systematically improving city, state and national overall health. This research is part of a large federal, state and local government 'healthy communities' partnership that is using an evidence-based strategy to positively target systems of health and ill health. An association was found, for example, between lack of access to fruit and vegetables and obesity, but this result does not necessarily mean that lack of access to fruit and vegetables causes obesity. There may actually be a lack of fruit and vegetables in an area due to a lack of demand for it, and this lack of demand might be a result of a causal factor that *also* contributes towards obesity — such as low economic status.

Conclusion

Now that you know at least something about the nature of inferential statistics, hypothesis testing, statistical significance, effect size, confidence intervals and experimental design, we can now move on to discuss some particularly commonly used, useful and health-science–relevant statistical tests in the following chapters.

Quick reference summary

- If a statistical test leads to a statistically significant result, we can infer that our sample result is true of our populations of interest, and is not just true of our sample.

- We need to know whether our results are meaningful as well as statistically significant, which in the area of health-science research often means *clinically meaningful.*

- Confidence intervals allow us to make more expansive interpretations of our results than do measures of statistical significance.

- Some major types of experimental design include the fully experimental, the quasi-experimental, the observational and the correlational. These designs differ in the extent of causal relationship that exists between conditions and outcomes.

References

1. Gruska M, Gaul G, Winkler M, et al. Increased occurrence of out-of-hospital cardiac arrest on Mondays in a community-based study. *Chronobiology International.* 2005;22(1):107-120.

2. Clarke MS, Wills RA, Bowman RV, et al. Exploratory study of the 'weekend effect' for acute medical admissions to public hospitals in Queensland, Australia. *Internal Medicine Journal.* 2010;40(11):777-783.

3. Kirsch I, Deacon BJ, Huedo-Medina TB, et al. Initial severity and antidepressant benefits: a meta-analysis of data submitted to the food and drug administration. *PLOS Medicine.* 2008;5:260–268.

4. Möller HJ. Isn't the efficacy of antidepressants clinically relevant? A critical comment on the results of the metaanalysis by Kirsch et al. 2008. *European Archives of Psychiatry and Clinical Neuroscience.* 2008;258(8):451-455.

5. Maxwell S, Delaney H. *Designing Experiments and Analyzing Data.* Mahwah, NJ: Lawrence Erlbaum Associates; 2004.

6. Valsiner J. Integrating psychology within the globalizing world: a requiem to the post-modernist experiment with Wissenschaft. *Integrated Psychological Behavior Science.* 2009;43(1):1-21.

7. Vitale AT, O'Connor PC. The effect of Reiki on pain and anxiety in women with abdominal hysterectomies: a quasi-experimental pilot study. *Holistic Nursing Practice.* 2006;20(6):263-272.

8. Lebeau M, Mathoulin-Pélissier S, Bellera C, et al. Breast cancer care compared with clinical guidelines: an observational study in France. *BMC Public Health.* 2011;11(Jan. 20):45.

CHAPTER 7

MEASURES OF DIFFERENCES 1: T-TESTS AND THE CHI-SQUARE TEST

Dean McKenzie and Stephen McKenzie

OBJECTIVES

After carefully reading this chapter you will discover:

- the principles underlying measures of differences
- what a t-test is, and how this differs from a chi-square test
- what a chi-square test is, and how this differs from a t-test
- a cure for disunity.

Introduction

A common principle of statistics, and also of life, is that things are often *different* from other things (as well as often being *associated* with other things, which we will cover in Chapters 9 and 10). You might have already discovered just how much things, and people, can differ, according to characteristics such as gender, age, intelligence, diagnosis or football team supported, or all of these characteristics. In this chapter and Chapter 8, we will provide you with ways of formally testing these differences.

No matter what interests you professionally or personally, there will be times when it is important for you to know just how real or true the apparent differences in your phenomena of interest are. A very famous psychology professor was once inspired to develop an important psychological theory when he got sick after eating bearnaise sauce.[1] This sickness was possibly due to dodgy egg yolk rather than to the shallot or the tarragon contained in the dish, but for years afterwards he could not eat bearnaise sauce, perhaps unconsciously assuming that it makes people sick. It is always hard to work with n = 1, but obviously there are unlikely to be true population differences between the bilious effects of bearnaise sauce versus those of other sauces, such as bechamel. The famous professor's adverse bearnaise reaction may have just been the (bad) luck of the culinary draw, rather than reflecting an actual difference between the entire population of bearnaise sauces versus the entire population of bechamel sauces.

You might be professionally or personally motivated even sooner than you anticipate to objectively test whether or not two or more sets of measurements are truly different from one another, in the sense that they come from populations with different characteristics, such as populations with different means. We will therefore provide you with the methods to calculate these differences, and the principles to understand what you are doing, by introducing you in this chapter to some of the best-known, best-loved and most useful statistical techniques in the statistical pantheon — the t-test and the chi-square test. The t-test allows us to test the statistical significance of differences between two arithmetic means and the chi-square test allows us to test the statistical significance of differences between two or more groups of frequencies. We will introduce you to the analysis of variance (ANOVA) in the chapter 8, and this will allow you to compare differences between more than two means.

The t-test

There are many situations in which it is important for us to know whether the apparent differences between two sets of phenomena reflect actual differences in the populations from which the samples are presumably drawn. For example, we might be trialling a new drug or therapy and be interested in whether or not it works. We can use the t-test to tell us whether the mean score on a dependent variable, such as general health or perceived quality of life, differs in the populations from which our post-intervention and pre-intervention groups were drawn. We can also compare the means of two unrelated groups of scores, such as the quality-of-life measures of migrant and locally born women who have recently had a baby. This is an actual research and clinical study that was recently reported by the Department of Health Sciences at La Trobe University, Melbourne. The study showed no statistically significant differences between migrant and locally born women who had just had a baby on outcomes such as depression and perceived acceptable level of life satisfaction.[2]

We can also use the t-test to tell us whether scores on a dependent variable, such as general health or quality of life, are *significantly* higher in one group than they are in the other group, although it must always be kept in mind that statistical significance does not mean practical or clinical significance. With sufficiently large samples, a mean of 10.2 can be significantly higher than a mean of 10.1, in a statistical sense. Such a finding would just indicate, however, that the chance of incorrectly rejecting the null hypothesis of no difference between populations (that is, that the populations have identical means, such as 10.1 and 10.1), when in fact the null hypothesis is false, is less than or equal to 5%, or 0.05.

The t-test can also be used to compare a single set of scores with hypothetical underlying population scores, such as the mean score on a measure of health-related quality of life in a psychiatric inpatient ward compared with the mean score for the whole hospital.

In this chapter we will present a general t-test training example that involves comparing characteristics of supporters of two different Australian Rules football clubs, and also a real-research health-related example that involves comparing the effectiveness of two Alzheimer's disease drug treatments. The same underlying principles apply to any comparisons that you might be interested in making, and we will start you off in a safe statistical harbour where you can develop your basic statistical seaworthiness before setting off in search of even more significant adventure on the statistical high seas. We will provide a worked training example for the paired samples t-test only, because this is easier to compute by hand and understand than the two-sample or independent samples t-test, which would be used to compare two independent groups, such as males and females.

Underlying principles and assumptions

No matter how many or what kinds of score sets your research question requires, the basic principle underlying t-tests remains the same — and is also the same as the principle underlying the analysis of variance (ANOVA) (discussed in Chapter 8), for the t-test can be seen as a special case of

Box 7.1 **Setting the statistical scene**

The eminent chemist and statistician William Sealy Gosset (1876–1937) was born in Canterbury, England, and worked for many years at the Guinness brewery in Dublin before eventually rising to anonymous fame as the 'Student' who devised what is now known as Student's t-test. Student's t-test is a statistical method that uses probability theory to inform us about whether the mean of one set of scores is truly different from the mean of another set of scores, in the sense that they reflect true differences in the populations from which the samples were drawn.

William Gosset's invention of the t-test meant that statistics could thereafter be applied to an increasingly broad range of real-world applications, such as brewing better beer. Fortunately for the invention of the t-test, beer-brewing research is mainly concerned with the testing of small samples (that is, fewer than 20 or so observations), so it was a practical imperative for Gosset to devise a statistical means of allowing for small samples and therefore allowing valid inferences to be made from them. The rest is statistical history.

Having published under the pseudonym 'Student', Gosset was not directly honoured for his enormous contribution to statistical science, unlike Pascal, Galton and Pearson. Although statistical veneration eluded him in his lifetime, Gosset did manage eventually to achieve the rank of chief brewer at Guinness's new brewery in London.

ANOVA. The principle is that both these measures of differences use formulas that resemble signal-to-noise ratios: they provide proportions of variance between groups (signal) to variance between individual cases (noise, or error). You could even see this as a sausage-to-sizzle ratio, or Guinness-to-froth ratio, if you prefer, where the sausage and the Guinness correspond to the 'signal' and the sizzle and the froth correspond to the 'noise'. These tests allow us to transform sets of scores into single variance ratio values, and then obtain the statistical significance of differences between means — represented by p-values.

The t-test and its nonparametric equivalents, which will be defined and described below, provide us with measures of the differences between two means, which can then be converted into a level of statistical significance. These tests constitute particular and commonly used examples of the general inferential statistical procedure that was described in Chapter 5. It is important in applying these tests to calculate the confidence intervals and to consider the effect sizes that were described in Chapter 6, as well as to consider the level of statistical significance. The application of the confidence interval to the t-test can give us useful information, including:

- the range of differences between our two sample means that we are confident, at a specified confidence level (95%), are true of the underlying populations.

- more specific information about confidence intervals (as described further on, in 'Beyond Statistical Significance').

Confidence-interval information is an important addition to the basic information that we obtain from a t-test, including the probability that a difference between two means as large as or larger than the one we observed could have arisen by chance if the null hypothesis of no difference between the population means was in fact true. Considering only statistical significance, rather than the broader information that our data can provide, is similar to making important legal decisions based only on circumstantial evidence.

Before we can appropriately apply any t-test we need to ensure that our data meet the t-test's assumptions of being sampled from normally distributed populations and measured on an interval or ratio scale (see Chapter 2). If we have ordinal data or if we have interval or ratio data that do not come from normally distributed populations, we may be able to use a nonparametric t-test equivalent.

As with so many things in life and statistics, there are many different definitions of *parametric* versus *nonparametric*. This brief definition is based on one given in a classic text on nonparametric statistics.[3] Parametric tests require the data to have been sampled from a population with a specified probability distribution, such as the normal distribution. The t-test is an example of a parametric test. Nonparametric tests make more general assumptions of the data than parametric tests and do not require the population probability distribution to be completely specified. Examples of nonparametric tests include the Wilcoxon-Mann-Whitney tests (described under 'Nonparametric t-test equivalents').

Before we apply either a t-test or a nonparametric equivalent, we also need to ensure that our data meet the assumption of independence of observations, which means not using data that have all been obtained from a common source, such as the same lemonade stand or even from a very large family, or several families. If we were to use such data, we would have something that statisticians call clustered data and we would have to use special techniques that are too complex to discuss here.[4]

Degrees of freedom

After we have calculated a t-test, we need to compare our obtained t-value with a critical level of t to find out if it is significant, and to do this we need to use 'degrees of freedom', rather than N (number of cases). 'Degrees of freedom' is not actually a statistical term that conveniently quantifies an important measure of quality of life, but it may be even more computationally useful. It is not necessary to have a comprehensive understanding of the mathematical basis of degrees of freedom, but it will help your statistical literacy and inform your readings of computer output or t-value tables if you know something about their underlying principles.

Degrees of freedom is a mathematical principle that is used to obtain the statistical significance level (p) that relates to particular values such as t-values. There are several formulas for calculating degrees of freedom, including n − 1 for paired-samples t-tests, where n is the total number of pairs in our sample. For an independent samples t-test, we use:

$$(n1-1)+(n2-1)$$

where n1 is the total number of observations in our first sample of scores and n2 is the total number of observations in our second group of scores.

To illustrate the underlying principle of degrees of freedom, consider a scenario where we are interested in three numbers — 5, 7 and 9 — and the mean of these numbers is 7. Our mathematical mission is to change any of the numbers without changing the mean. How many of these three numbers can we change without changing the mean? In this case, we are free to vary only two of the numbers (three, or the total number of numbers, minus one) if we are to keep the mean constant, and you are welcome to try this experiment for yourselves if you are not yet convinced.

T-tests and z-tests

The *t-test* provides us with a standard score, comprising of the ratio of our between-groups variance to our within-groups variance. The t-test can be used to calculate a t-value, which we can then use as a special case of the normal probability distribution that we introduced in Chapters 3 and 5 — namely, the t-distribution — to express the level of differences between sets of scores in terms of a probability that the observed or larger difference between the means could have arisen by chance. If this probability is less than or equal to our designated critical level, such as 0.05, then the difference is deemed statistically significant, although this is not necessarily practically or clinically significant. As mentioned in Chapter 6, 'statistical significance' just means that there is only a small probability that a difference in the underlying populations, no matter how tiny, has arisen by chance, if in fact the null hypothesis is true. 'Practical significance' or 'a clinically meaningful result' means that the difference is sufficiently large to be meaningful.

Closely related to the t-test is the *z-test*, which uses a similar formula to that used for the t-test. The z-test is used when the population standard deviation is known and when samples sizes are large enough. We virtually never know the population standard deviation, which is why we use inferential statistics to infer population characteristics from sample ones. The t-test is therefore far more generally used than the z-test, because the former uses the sample standard deviation rather than the population standard deviation and, vitally, can be used with small samples.

Types of t-test: when to use what?

If our research or personal interest involves finding out the significance of differences between two sets of related or unrelated scores, we can use a t-test to help us find an answer.

An independent-samples t-test is appropriate for comparing the means of two different samples such as males and females, or members of an experimental group administered a particular drug and members of a control group administered a placebo, or 'sugar pill'. Examples of independent-samples t-tests in action are provided below in 'T-tests in Action'.

A paired-samples t-test is appropriate for comparing the means of a group that was measured twice, or two separate groups that were matched on variables such as age and gender and are therefore related. Please do not worry unduly if you have only one group of scores, because there is also a one-sample t-test, which assesses the statistical significance of difference between the mean of a group of scores and the mean of a population. This test uses the same formula as the paired-samples t-test, except that the latter uses differences between means obtained from two sets of scores, such as those from a group of people measured before and after a particular event taking place. Examples of paired samples t-tests in action are provided below.

Before we can calculate any t-test, we need to start with a basis of comparison between our groups of scores. This is our measure, our dependent variable. We can then apply a t-test to the scores on our measure to calculate whether the observed differences between groups on it are statistically significant, reflecting actual differences in the populations. It is also important that our results are real, such as really clinically meaningful: you were introduced to the importance of effect size in Chapter 6, and we will return to it in Chapter 12.

T-tests in action: general

A general example of how to choose an appropriate t-test to help us answer a research question begins with our research and clinical interest in whether supporters of one Australian Rules football team are more obnoxious than supporters of another football team, or even if their level of obnoxiousness can be reduced. Perhaps we have a grant to investigate this phenomenon, or perhaps we have a grudge, or perhaps we are just curious. Unfortunately there is no currently available football-supporter obnoxiousness scale to use as our dependent variable that meets our rigorous criteria for validity and reliability, so we need to devise one. We therefore painstakingly produce the soon-to-be-widely-used football supporter obnoxiousness scale — 'verbal abuse per instance of dialogue' (VAPID) scale — and attend some conveniently located football games to collect some data. Our innovative research project is probably more likely to get us into the papers or a hospital than onto the Nobel prize short list, but sometimes research can be deeply rather than superficially satisfying.

Which type of t-test we need to apply to our research data depends on how we have constructed our research design, and on what data we have collected. We can measure the same group of football supporters twice and then calculate how different their mean scores are between testings, which means that we will need to use a paired-samples t-test. An example of this test would be applying VAPID to the supporters of a particular football team before they are given an intervention designed to improve their verbal behaviour — such as an alcohol restriction — and then testing them again afterwards. We can therefore test a research hypothesis that the intervention is effective. If our research question involves comparing the means of two different groups of people, we will need to use an independent-samples t-test. A general example of this type of t-test consists of administering the VAPID to supporters of two rival football teams, to test the hypothesis that one team's supporters are more verbally abusive than the other team's supporters. This hypothesis might be based on our preliminary research, or on our life experience, or a hunch.

An example of the use of a one-sample t-test would be in a situation where, perhaps unsurprisingly, we have only one sample of data, and we would like to use our single data sample to test a research hypothesis. In this case we can use a one-sample t-test to compare our single-sample data mean with the statistical equivalent to a par in golf — a hypothetical population mean.

T-tests in action: health-related

A health-related example of choosing an appropriate t-test begins with our research interest in whether a new drug purported to improve the symptoms of Alzheimer's disease (AD) is effective. We could use scores on a memory test as our dependent variable and administer this test to a group of patients with AD before and after they have been treated with the new drug. We could use a paired-samples t-test to test the hypothesis that the drug results in a statistically significant improvement on the same group of patients tested twice. It should be noted that the patients may recover in time without the drug (a 'maturation' effect in Campbell and Stanley's classic terminology[5]). This type of design can therefore be problematic, because we cannot be sure whether improvement is due to time or drug, and so it would be better to have two groups.[6]

A more comprehensive way of constructing our research question would consist of giving a new drug treatment to a group of patients with

Alzheimer's disease (AD) and giving a placebo to another group of AD patients, and then testing for differences (drug effect) between the drug-treated and placebo-treated groups We could also use a memory test as our dependent variable, and test our research question: does the intervention work better than a placebo? Because our research and clinical question in this case involves comparing the means of two different groups of people, it would be appropriate to use an independent-samples t-test, although in practice such designs are often handled with more sophisticated methods.[7,8]

Nonparametric t-test equivalents

Our research question might lead us to a situation where we have ordinal data (see Chapter 2) rather than interval or ratio data. Alternatively, we might have interval or ratio data but be concerned that the data contain some extreme scores, or are otherwise not assumed to have been sampled from populations that are normally distributed. This may mean that our data are nonparametric and therefore not suitable for application of the t-test, which is intended for parametric analyses. Fortunately, there are tests specifically intended for these data, collectively known (logically enough) as nonparametric tests.

The Wilcoxon test was invented by Frank Wilcoxon (1892–1965), who first described it in a paper that he published in 1945. Like Gosset, Wilcoxon was a chemist and statistician, but he worked primarily for the American Cyanamid Company (known for making polio vaccine as well as for a famous brand of aftershave and various other useful products). Wilcoxon's test can be regarded as a nonparametric analogue or equivalent of the Student's t-test, and is basically exactly the same as the Mann-Whitney test, which was published by Henry Berthold Mann (1905–2000) and his student Donald Ransom Whitney (1915–2001) in 1947. These tests are sometimes collectively described as Wilcoxon-Mann-Whitney tests. The rank-sum version is appropriate for comparing differences between scores from two independent groups, and the signed-rank version for analysing differences between scores from paired samples.

These tests are conceptually related to the more commonly used nonparametric correlation statistics (discussed in Chapter 9) and are based on a similar underlying principle of conversion of raw scores into rank values. This process may also help to reduce problems associated with extreme scores, or outliers, which you may remember from Chapter 3, in that the Wilcoxon-Mann-Whitney tests are employed to compare the means of the ranked observations rather than the means of the actual observations. The Wilcoxon-Mann-Whitney tests do not assume that the data are normally distributed; they are suitable for application to ordinal data and can generally handle outliers better than t-tests can. In our previous football team and Alzheimer's examples, if our VAPID or AD-related memory scores had been measured on an ordinal scale such as a Likert scale (where responses are scored, for example, with VAPID scores from 1 = no verbal abuse, to 7 = incessant verbal abuse; or with AD scores from 1 = mild AD, to 3 = severe AD), then it would be appropriate to use a Mann-Whitney-Wilcoxon test rather than a t-test. (For more information about the Wilcoxon test, refer to Corder and Foreman,[9] and Siegel and Castellan.[3])

Many health-science researchers and clinicians use t-tests and other parametric tests on Likert scale data. This practice is not technically correct, but seems to be undertaken on the basis of tradition, especially in psychology.[3] The Wilcoxon-Mann-Whitney family of tests do not require the same level of statistical inquisition of our data as the t-test, but still assume independence of observations and also that the samples have both come from populations of the same and symmetric shape and so have equivalent variance. If our data violate the latter assumption, no doubt innocently, then we can use a special type of t-test (if other assumptions are met, and we have two groups of people) known as the independent-samples t-test with separate variance estimate, or we can use more complex parametric and nonparametric tests, as described by Wilcox.[10]

Calculating t-tests

In our increasingly computer driven age we are often quite happy to allow our high-tech slaves — our computers — to do our hard mental labour for us, and this includes hard statistical labour. Most reputable computers will run t-tests and other statistics for us until the cows come home, if we instruct them to do so, but they do not generally explain to us afterwards what they have done, or why. It might not seem all that likely that one day you will end up stranded on a desert island without a computer or a power point to plug it into and are desperately craving some 'survival' statistics (such as on comparing the negative effects of one potentially poisonous foodstuff or water supply with another) and so will urgently need to calculate a t-test. Knowing how to calculate a t-test without a computer, however, is a very useful skill, even if you never end up stuck on a desert island without computer access. This is because learning how to calculate even one type of t-test will help you to understand the principles that underlie a whole family of statistics — measures of differences — which include t-tests and ANOVAs.

A practical as well as theoretical understanding of t-tests will help you not only to appropriately perform a wide range of useful statistical tests, but also to understand what you are doing, as well as why you are doing it. Researchers or clinicians who are completely computer-reliant, and cannot understand the inner workings of even a simple t-test task, are somewhat related to builders who are so nail-gun reliant that they cannot understand the inner workings of even a simple nail-hammering task. Learning the statistical analysis ropes is therefore like learning enough about our car to cope if something goes wrong with it, by being, for example, able to check its oil levels rather than having to call in a mechanic (although obviously it is very often appropriate to call in the experts, whether mechanical or statistical).

It is now time to embark on the exciting statistical adventure of working out a t-test (paired samples) for yourself, step by step, as this (along with the one-sample t-test that shares the same formula) is the easiest t-test to calculate by hand and is a good t-test training example.

Calculating a paired-samples (or matched-samples) t-test

An interesting recent example of health-related statistics in action involves the clinical trial in Iran of a commonly available herb for the treatment of Alzheimer's disease. This genuine and real-world international research example can be used to demonstrate the workings of a t-test, and may even inspire you to undertake your own research into something that particularly interests you.

Researchers at the Tehran University of Medical Sciences conducted a randomised and placebo-controlled trial of the rare and expensive spice saffron as a non-toxic, non-invasive, non-drug-company-profitable and commonly available intervention for improving AD symptoms.[11] They administered saffron to mild and moderate AD patients, and then examined post-treatment improvement of symptom levels, using a cognitive function test and a clinical dementia rating scale as their dependent variables. The results of this study showed that AD patients treated with saffron for 16 weeks did better than controls on a test of cognitive function. A paired-samples t-test could be used to compare the statistical significance of pre- versus post-saffron treatment in cognitive function scores in either one of the mild or moderate AD patient groups.

The first thing that we will need to do before we calculate a t-test is to choose the appropriate one to calculate. We know from the above discussion that the appropriate t-test for this example is a paired-samples t-test, because we are testing the same group of people twice. As ever, the first thing that we need to do is to get properly acquainted with our data, such as by checking the assumptions that we mentioned above, including calculating and examining its frequency distributions.

The paired-sample (or matched-sample) t-test formula is just the one-sample t-test formula applied to the differences between two sets of paired scores, and consists of:

$$t = \frac{Dmean - 0}{SE}$$

where $Dmean = \dfrac{\Sigma D}{n}$, $SE = \dfrac{DSD}{\sqrt{n}}$ and

$$DSD = \frac{\sqrt{\Sigma i - 1(D - Dmean)^2}}{n - 1}$$

This can be translated into English, or something closely resembling it, as:

> To calculate the difference between the means of two sets of scores, where these scores consist of measures of the same or a matched group, first find the mean of all of the difference scores between measure 1 and measure 2. Then divide this mean by the standard error of the mean difference between measure 1 and measure 2 scores. Note that the 0 in the top line refers to the expected differences between the underlying population means of the two groups if the null hypothesis (no difference between the groups) is true: in other words, under the null hypothesis, of no difference between pre- and post-saffron in regard to cognitive function.

We can divide our worked example of this into the following steps, based on a small, simulated sample, randomly generated so as to have similar characteristics to the published saffron study results:

1. *Generate an experimental hypothesis that we will statistically test, in this case that there will be a statistically significant difference in memory performance pre- and post-saffron administration. The null hypothesis is that there will be no such difference.*

2. *Calculate the mean of the differences in group scores between measure 1 and measure 2 (Table 7.1).*

This then gives us the answer to the top line of the formula:

$$\text{Dmean} - 0 = 2.30$$

Remember that 0 is the value expected under the null hypothesis of no difference in the means of the pre-test and post-test population scores.

3. *Calculate the standard error of the mean difference between t1 and t2 scores:*

   a. *Calculate the standard deviation of the difference scores, D, by adding up the squared deviations from the mean and then dividing by n (the number of pairs) minus one. This gives the variance. Taking the square root of the variance gives the standard deviation.*

$$\frac{64.10}{10-1} = \sqrt{7.12} = 2.67$$

   b. *Divide the standard deviation of the difference scores by the square root of n to calculate the standard error:*

$$\frac{2.67}{\sqrt{10}} = 0.84$$

TABLE 7.1 COGNITIVE FUNCTIONS SCORES, PRE- AND POST-SAFFRON TREATMENT

Participant	Pre-saffron	Post-saffron	Difference (D) (between post- and pre-saffron)	$(D - Dmean)^2$
1	7	9	2	0.09
2	5	9	4	2.89
3	6	4	-2	18.49
4	4	7	3	0.49
5	9	12	3	0.49
6	9	10	1	1.69
7	11	11	0	5.29
8	7	8	1	1.69
9	8	11	3	0.49
10	5	13	8	32.49
Mean	7.10	9.40	2.30	64.10 (Sum)
SD	2.18	2.63	2.67	

4. *Divide the answer to the top line of the t-test formula (i.e. the mean of the differences) by the answer to the bottom line (i.e. the standard error):*

$$t = \frac{2.30}{0.84} = 2.74$$

5. *Look up 2.74 in a t-table (such as in Howell[16]) at n − 1 degrees of freedom.*

Our degrees of freedom in this situation are n − 1. Remember that we use degrees of freedom rather than n to calculate the significance of statistical tests such as a paired-samples t-test because this takes the principles we described above into account. In our t-test calculation we obtained our sample variance by calculating deviations from the sample mean. The sum of deviations about the mean is always zero, and so only n − 1 deviations are free to vary. If, for example, n is 7, we need to know only 6 of the variations from the mean to calculate the seventh.

To be statistically significant at the 0.05 level (for a two-tailed test, which is appropriate when we do not nominate an expected direction of difference) with 9 degrees of freedom (in this case 10 pairs minus 1), our obtained t must be greater than or equal to 2.26 (which it is), so we can reject our null hypothesis of no difference between the population means for pre- and post-test scores. To be statistically significant at the 0.01 level for a two-tailed test with 9 degrees of freedom, our obtained t must be greater than or equal to 3.25, which it is not. Therefore, our result is statistically significant only at the 0.05 level, which means (unless we have a reason for using 0.01) that we can reject the null hypothesis of no difference between pre- and post-treatment scores.

Beyond statistical significance

Because our t-test result is statistically significant, we can presume that the underlying population difference is unlikely to be zero, but what actually is the population difference? We might like to say that we are pretty sure that the true or population difference ranges between x and y. However 'pretty sure' is not generally regarded within polite statistical society as being a sufficiently specific description, so it is far better for us to be able to say that we are 95% confident that the true or population difference value ranges between x and y. As you may remember from Chapter 6, a 95% confidence interval between x and y simply indicates that, if we generate an infinite or at least a very large number of samples of size n and work out the confidence interval, 95% of them will contain the true population value. In order to achieve 95% confidence, we will need to calculate a 95% confidence interval, which in the case of a paired-sample t-test is:

> D (for mean of differences) plus or minus (multiplier times the standard error)

For small samples, our multiplier will be based on the t distribution. We have already obtained the critical value of t for a two-tailed test (at an alpha of 0.05 and at 9 degrees of freedom) of 2.26 in our saffron example. This means that 95% of the values in a t distribution for 9 degrees of freedom will range between −2.26 and 2.26. The lower limit of the confidence interval for the true or population difference is therefore 2.30 (mean of differences) minus 2.26 times the standard error of 0.84 = 2.30 minus 1.90 = 0.40. The upper limit is 2.30 plus 2.26 times 0.84, which equals 2.30 plus 1.90 = 4.20. Thus we can be 95% confident that our true or population mean difference in this situation ranges between 0.40 and 4.20, which is quite a broad difference. This is similar to a real-life situation in which we are told by our mechanic that it will cost somewhere between $40 and $420 to fix our car's brakes, or by our dentist that it will cost somewhere between $40 and $420 to fix a tooth.

Our t-test analysis has provided us with a result which has led us to reject our null hypothesis that saffron does not improve AD symptoms, and we can perhaps now throw a party to celebrate, if we consider our *t*-value and research incidentals budget to be large enough to justify it. However tempted we may be to celebrate a statistically significant result, we need to soberly consider our broader statistical situation, including the clinical significance of our results. The statistical significance of this particular result merely means that the population mean difference (pre- to post-saffron treatment) memory score is unlikely to be zero, but this difference may be trivial and not justify clinical implications such as recommending that saffron treatment for AD be adopted, even if it is inexpensive and has few side effects.

Before we celebrate any statistical results, no matter how apparently exciting they may be, we need to consider their other attributes, including their clinical significance. This can be measured by calculating effect size (covered in more detail in Chapters 6 and 12). There are several ways to construct an effect size for a paired-samples t-test,[12] and we can construct a measure of effect size in our saffron treatment example simply by dividing the mean difference of 2.30 by the pre-test standard deviation, which is 2.30 divided by 2.18 = 1.06. Therefore, saffron appears to have an overall effect of 1.06 pre-test standard deviations, which according to the arbitrary but conventionally employed criteria outlined by Jacob Cohen, would be a large effect.[13] For t-tests, Cohen suggested that effects should be at least 0.80 for a large effect, 0.50 for a medium effect, and 0.20 for a small effect.

An Australian health-science example

A real-research example of a paired-samples t-test (and a chi-square test) in action is provided by a study of access to hospital care of Australian emergency department (ED) patients'.[14] This study investigated changes to access block in a 4-year period. ('Access block' has been defined as the inability of potential ED patients to get proper access to hospital care, which in Australia is defined as an ED wait of more than 8 hours.) On the basis of paired-samples t-test (and chi-square test results), the researchers demonstrated that around one-third of all patients receiving ED care experienced access block, and it was concluded that most Australian hospitals are inefficient, if efficiency is interpreted as resulting in low rates of access block.

Epilogue for t-test

We could also use our Iranian saffron AD treatment example to demonstrate how to calculate a one-sample t-test and an independent-samples t-test, but there is no need to add to your computational t-test training load. The basic principles underlying the calculation of measures of difference are similar, no matter what their particular formulaic manifestation. The active ingredient of a t-test, whether applied to saffron treatments or to the VAPID scale or to anything else, is that it provides a statistic which is a ratio of signal (differences between our sets or groups of interests) to noise (differences within our sets or groups of interest).

The saffron example illustrates the principles common to many statistical tests of differences between sets or groups. To compare a saffron-treated

AD group and a placebo-treated control group, rather than the saffron-treated AD group pre- and post-treatment, we would use an independent-samples rather than a paired-samples t-test. To make both of these comparisons (to compare two or more groups on pre- and post-treatment scores) in the same analysis, or to compare more than two groups of scores in any situation, we will need to step up from a t-test to an ANOVA, which will be covered in Chapter 8.

Comparing counts: the chi-square test

Disinformation could be said to be spreading even more rapidly in our modern world that it ever did, and it is getting increasingly easier to involuntarily catch disinformation overload from outlets such as the mass media. A hypothetical example of our real disinformation epidemic starts with the typical 'statistic' that an 'alarming' 2.3% of the population of Manangatang have presented to their local emergency department with an alcohol or other drug-related (AOD) condition in the last 12 months. Such statistical scariness is designed to attract attention and therefore sell newspapers or otherwise increase media profitability. The damage that this can cause to people who are not statistically literate enough to be protected from such brazen misuse of statistics is potentially enormous. The intention of the disinformation pushers in this particular example is to scare people into assuming that AOD-related harm in their area is obviously rampant and getting worse, and influence them to buy more newspapers or watch more TV news to keep 'informed' about it.

Statistical literacy can protect us from disinformation by encouraging us to ask relevant questions, such as 'What should I compare such percentages to?', and therefore 'What's the baseline rate of alcohol-related hospital admissions in Manangatang?' We need to know the answers to these questions to know whether rate of AOD-related ED admissions is actually worse than it usually is, or is the same, or better. We should also ask whether there has been some special event in Manangatang in the last 12 months that has artificially and temporarily increased AOD-related hospital admissions, such as the 25th anniversary reunion of the Manangatang Statistician's Guild (MSG).

There are several appropriate methods for comparing proportions, such as the binomial test, odds ratio, relative risk and the chi-square test.[9,16] We will cover odds ratios and relative risks in more detail in Chapter 12, but will introduce you to the chi-square test here because it is widely used. It also has the advantage that it can be used when there are more than two groups, or more than two outcomes, but we will restrict ourselves to discussing the simple two (rows or groups) by two (columns or outcomes) design here.

Karl (born Carl) Pearson was a nineteenth-century English statistician who gave the world many important statistical tests. You will learn more

---

Box 7.2 **Par for a statistical course**

What our modern world perhaps needs even more than another information superhighway lane is the statistical information equivalent to a par in golf — a method for comparing a baseline or expected value with an actual or obtained value. In golf a score is not presented as a raw score, such as 125, because unless we know a lot of other things that raw score does not tell us anything useful. A golfer's score is presented instead in terms of shots above or below par. Par is an expected value, the number of shots that a competent and sober golfer would normally be expected to take to play a hole. The golfer's score is therefore expressed as a number of shots above par (bad) or below par (good).

The par principle has found its way into English colloquial language, such as when one is feeling 'below par' (actually an inaccurate borrowing from golfing language, because this should be a good thing). Comparison of observed with expected values is also the basis of scoring in one-day cricket matches using the Duckworth-Lewis method[15] (now widely used to provide arbitrated results of washed-out cricket games), in which a team's score is based on a par, or expected value, by relating it to the results of many other matches.

---

about him in Chapter 9 as the developer of the Pearson's correlation coefficient. Pearson also gave us a very useful and widely used nonparametric statistical test that allows us to calculate the proportion of actual to expected scores, and the significance of the differences of proportions and frequencies. This is known as the chi-square test.

The chi-square test that we are presenting here is the type intended for two-way tables — for example, gender by diagnosis, or rurality (Mentone, Manangatang) by hospital admission. Each variable can have two or more possible levels (for example, four different diagnostic categories) but there should be only two variables.

A chi-square test example

Imagine that we have a professional or personal interest in whether there is a difference in AOD-related hospital admissions relating to the playing activities of two sporting teams — the deep-country-based Manangatang Football Team and the deep-city-based Mentone Football Team. Our interest might be professional, in that we might have a grant to find out whether there is, as every country person knows, more AOD-related harm in the city, or as every city person knows, more AOD-related harm in the country. Our interest might be personal, in that we might want to know which place to avoid. The first thing that we will need to do to statistically satisfy our research curiosity is to think of a way of measuring our research interest. We will therefore define our dependent variable as the proportion of AOD-related to non-AOD-related hospital emergency department admissions in Manangatang and Mentone after home football games.

We would ideally compare our characteristics of interest between an overall urban sample and an overall rural sample, as there may be other differences between Manangatang and Mentone apart from one being metropolitan and one being rural. For example, they may happen to differ in gender composition or in number of hotels per head of population, but we will conveniently assume for our chi-square example that the only difference between Manangatang and Mentone is that one is in the city and the other in the country (but please do not make this assumption when working without the safety net of a fictitious chi-square calculation example).

The formula for calculating a chi-square is:

$$\chi^2 = \frac{\Sigma(O - E)^2}{E}$$

where E = the row total multiplied by the column total divided by the total N. This can be translated into English, or something pretty close to it, as:

To obtain a measure of the difference between counts obtained from two separate groups, add up the differences between the actual observed counts and the counts expected under the null hypothesis, after having squared these differences to eliminate negative values, and divide the squared difference by the expected difference.

We can divide a worked example of this into the four following steps:

1. *Generate an experimental hypothesis that we will statistically test, in this case that there will be a significant difference in the proportion of alcohol-related emergency hospital admissions between the Manangatang Maulers and the Mentone Marauders when each team plays at home. The null hypothesis is that there will be no such difference.*

2. *Create a table of the alcohol-related and non-alcohol-related frequencies for Manangatang and Mentone hospital admissions when the Maulers and Marauders are playing at home (Table 7.2).*

Note that for smaller samples designs such as this one — in this case, two (columns) by two (rows) — some statisticians suggest the use of a correction originally suggested by Sir Frank Yates (1902–94), who worked

TABLE 7.2   FREQUENCIES OF ALCOHOL-RELATED AND NON-ALCOHOL-RELATED HOSPITAL ED ATTENDANCES

	ED admissions		
	Non-alcohol-related	Alcohol-related	Total
Manangatang home games	328	75	403
Mentone home games	518	91	609
Total	846	166	N = 1012

with Sir Ronald Fisher at the Rothamsted Experimental Station in England and later became the head of statistics there. Current thinking, however, appears to be that Yates's correction for continuity, which involves subtracting 0.5 from the difference between observed and expected frequencies before squaring them, is too conservative. In practice, computers offer other solutions to this potential problem, including 'Fisher's exact tests' or 'permutation tests'.[16,17] These tests are, however, difficult, if not impossible, to do by hand, so we will leave them alone and mention them briefly again in Chapter 14.

3. *Work out the squared differences between our observed and expected values, and then divide the expected values for each cell and add these results together:*

$$\chi^2 = \frac{(328-336.90)^2}{336.90} + \frac{(75-66.10)^2}{66.10}$$
$$+ \frac{(518-509.10)^2}{509.10} + \frac{(91-99.90)^2}{99.90}$$
$$\chi^2 = 0.23 + 1.20 + 0.16 + 0.79$$
$$\chi^2 = 2.38$$

4. *Using a table of the chi-square distribution, which can be readily found in many more detailed statistics texts,[3,9,16] we then compare 2.38 with the critical level for degrees of freedom of 1, where the degrees of freedom are the number of rows minus one multiplied by the number of columns minus one, and we find a critical value of 3.84 (this critical value applies for any two-by-two table, with alpha = 0.05). Our obtained chi-square of 2.38 does not equal or exceed this value and so we cannot reject our null hypothesis that there is no statistically significant difference between the proportion of alcohol-related emergency department admissions in Manangatang and Mentone on home football game days.*

We can therefore walk the streets of either Manangatang or Mentone on a home football game day equally content or discontent in the knowledge that our chances of experiencing an alcohol-related emergency department hospital admission are no higher or lower than they would be in the other place.

We will return to the two-by-two tables that we used in this chapter to illustrate chi-square in Chapter 12, where we cover odds ratios and relative risk with an example that compares the risk of having a heart attack when taking aspirin to the risk of having a heart attack when not taking aspirin. These are very important health-science statistical techniques and, unlike chi-square tests, also readily allow confidence intervals to be calculated.

Conclusion

The exciting conclusion to 'Measures of differences' will be presented in Chapter 8, in which you will learn what you need to know, and possibly even more, about the ANOVA family of tests, which are underpinned by the same basic principles as t-tests, but can be applied to more interesting situations.

Quick reference summary

- A common principle of statistics and also of life is that things are often *different* from other things, and t-tests can help us to measure these differences.

- To calculate t-tests, we use formulas that resemble signal-to-noise ratios (or sausage-to-sizzle ratios). T-tests give us ratios of between-groups variance (signal) to between-cases variance (noise, or statistical error).

- There are paired-samples t-tests (the same people are measured twice); independent-samples t-tests (two groups of people are measured) and one-sample t-tests (one group of people is measured).

- There are nonparametric equivalents to the t-test, such as the Wilcoxon-Mann-Whitney tests, that are appropriate for use with ordinal data (and possibly, non-normally distributed interval or ratio data).

- The use of the chi-square test (and the one-sample t-test) resembles the use of the par in golf — it allows us to compare observed phenomena with expected benchmarks.

References

1. Seligman MEP, Hager JL. Psychological boundaries of learning. The sauce-béarnaise syndrome. *Psychology Today*. 1972;6:59-1, 84-87.

2. Bandyopadhyay M, Small R, Watson LF, et al. Life with a new baby: how do immigrant and Australian-born women's experiences compare? *Australian and New Zealand Journal of Public Health*. 2010;34(4):412-421.

3. Siegel S, Castellan NJ. *Nonparametric Statistics for the Behavioral Sciences*. 2nd ed. New York: McGraw-Hill; 1988.

4. Dupont W. *Statistical Modeling for Biomedical Researchers: a Simple Introduction to the Analysis of Complex Data*. 2nd ed. New York: Cambridge University Press; 2009.

5. Campbell DT, Stanley JC. *Experimental and Quasi-experimental Designs for Research*. Boston, MA: Houghton Mifflin; 1966.

6. Shadish WR, Cook TD, Campbell DT. *Experimental and Quasi-experimental Designs for Generalized Causal Inference*. 2nd ed. Boston, MA: Houghton Mifflin; 2001.

7. Twisk J, Proper K. Evaluation of the results of a randomized controlled trial: how to define changes between baseline and follow-up. *Journal of Clinical Epidemiology*. 2004;57:223-227.

8. Forbes AB, Carlin JB. 'Residual change' analysis is not equivalent to analysis of covariance. *Journal of Clinical Epidemiology*. 2005;58:540-541.

9. Corder GW, Foreman DI. *Nonparametric Statistics for Non-statisticians: a Step-by-step Approach*. Hoboken, NJ: Wiley; 2009.

10. Wilcox RR. *Introduction to Robust Estimation and Hypothesis Testing*. 3rd ed. San Diego, CA: Academic Press; 2012.

11. Akhondzadeh S, Shafiee-Sabet M, Harirchian MH, et al. Saffron in the treatment of patients with mild to moderate Alzheimer's disease: A 16-week, randomized and placebo-controlled trial. *Journal of Clinical Pharmacy and Therapeutics*. 2010;35(5):581-587.

12. Cumming G. *Understanding the New Statistics: Effect Sizes, Confidence Intervals, and Meta-analysis*. New York: Routledge; 2012.

13. Cohen, J. *Statistical Power Analysis for the Behavioral Sciences*. 2nd ed. Hillsdale, NJ: Erlbaum; 1988.

14. Richardson D, Kelly A, Kerr D. Prevalence of access block in Australia 2004–2008. *Emergency Medicine Australasia.* 2009;21:472-478.

15. Duckworth-Lewis.com. The Duckworth-Lewis Method. Available online at http://www.duckworth-lewis.com/. Accessed 21 September 2012.

16. Howell D. *Statistical Methods for Psychology.* 7th ed. Belmont, CA: Duxbury Press; 2010.

17. Higgins JJ. *Introduction to Modern Nonparametric Statistics.* Pacific Grove, CA: Brooks/Cole-Thomson; 2004.

CHAPTER 8

MEASURES OF DIFFERENCES 2: ANALYSIS OF VARIANCE (ANOVA)

The habit of analysis has a tendency to wear away the feelings.

JOHN STUART MILL (1806–73)

OBJECTIVES

After carefully reading this chapter you will understand:

- where and when and why to use an ANOVA
- how to distinguish the different types of ANOVAs, without a microscope
- the underlying principles of an ANOVA, and how they relate to those of other measures of differences
- how to separate information wheat from disinformation chaff.

Introduction

The ANOVA can be seen as an extension of the logic of t-tests, which test for the significance of differences between two sample means. The t-test is also an analysis of variance, in the sense that it calculates the ratio of variance between two sets of scores to variance within a set of scores, and this can be seen as a signal-to-noise ratio. The ANOVA allows us to do even more interesting things than t-tests allow us to do, by allowing us to test the statistical significance of differences between more than two sample means. This capacity is particularly useful in the health sciences because it is uncommon for health-science researchers and clinicians to be interested in the relationship between just two sets of scores, even though one of the most common health-science research designs, the randomised control trial (RCT), can be conducted with just two groups — a treatment group and a control. Health-science researchers, clinicians and other health professionals are usually interested in comparisons involving more than two conditions, such as at least two treatment conditions being compared with a control condition.

Comparisons involving more than two conditions can be made using ANOVA, as this very useful statistical tool allows comparisons that involve more than one condition of one independent variable, more than one independent variable, and even more than one dependent variable within a single analysis (see Chapter 2 for a description of variables). The ANOVA extends the logic and calculation characteristics of the t-test, so you do not need to learn ANOVA formulas or see a worked calculation example. Your hands-on experience in Chapter 7 of calculating a t-test and the ANOVA description provided in this chapter will equip you to run ANOVAs appropriately using a computer package (described in Chapter 14), and to interpret their output appropriately.

Underlying principles and assumptions

Principles

The basic computational principle that underlies ANOVA is the same as the basic principle that underlies t-tests. The measure of difference that it produces — in this case an F rather than a t — can be seen as a signal (between groups variance) to noise (within groups variance) ratio. As Fisher developed this test to assist with wheat yield analysis (Boxes 8.1 and 8.2), the ANOVA may even more appropriately be described as a wheat-to-chaff ratio. The defining difference between ANOVA and t-tests is that ANOVA allows us to calculate differences simultaneously between more than two groups of scores.

If we calculate an ANOVA or, far more likely, if we instruct our computer to calculate an ANOVA, there are assumptions of our data that

Box 8.1 **Statistics and purpose-built discovery**

The history of statistics is really the history of statistical problems and the innovative methodologies that statisticians have devised to overcome them. Problems associated with God, evolution, gambling, beer and wheat have led to the development of many of the most important advances in statistical science. This principle of purpose-built discovery is illustrated by the 'problem' of a falling apple (particularly problematic if it lands on you!) that inspired Newton to describe gravity. If Newton had not had a problem — an apple falling on him — he probably would not have bothered to discover, or at least to describe, an important principle that governs the actions of falling objects, including apples — the principle of gravity.

Bread is a human resource that is about as basic as apples, and it can be similarly scientifically inspirational. Bread, or actually the wheat that it is made from, is the stuff of statistics, as well as of other forms of life. The problem of how to produce more bread by increasing wheat yields inspired one of the great modern statistical developments. Sir Ronald Fisher was born in London in 1890 and died in Adelaide in 1962. As a young man, after turning down a statistics job offered by the great statistician Karl Pearson, he was given the highly statistically significant mission of analysing wheat yields. Fisher developed the ANOVA in response to the research needs of the Rothamsted Experimental Station in Hertfordshire, which was founded in 1843 and is the oldest agricultural research station in the world. The rest is statistical history.

it needs to meet. It is the responsibility of the researcher rather than of the researcher's statistical package to ensure that the analyses that are run via this medium are appropriate. Statistical packages merely follow our orders, good or bad, and we need sufficient general and analysis-specific statistical literacy to instruct them wisely and to interpret their output wisely. This principle relates to the development of good data sense, in that before we commence a meaningful analytical relationship with our data, such as by performing ANOVAs on it, we should first know it properly from having examined its characteristics via preliminary descriptive statistical analyses. These analyses provide us with important information, such as the nature of our data distribution and the possible existence of outliers.

> ### Box 8.2 **Development of the ANOVA**
>
> Sir Ronald Fisher built on the statistical work of Karl Pearson and William Gosset ('Student') by taking such concepts as the 'Student's' t and applying them to more complex data. Fisher, however, had a style and a genius of his own, which enabled him to develop a statistical method that was particularly well suited to the analysis of complex data. He took the statistical methodologies available to him further than they had ever been taken before, because he applied them to solving his own defining problems. These problems mainly concerned crop rotation, and to solve them he devised the analysis of variance (ANOVA) test to describe differences between more than two groups of scores, as well as relationships between them — interactions.
>
> Fisher also invented discriminant function analysis (perhaps on his days off), initiated the modern statistical usage of terms such as variance and randomisation, and established the distinction between *statistic,* meaning 'pertaining to a sample', and *parameter,* meaning 'pertaining to a population'. In case you were wondering, although Fisher invented the analysis of variance, the first person to call it ANOVA was the great American statistician John Tukey (1915–2000).

Assumptions

The ANOVA assumes that the variances of each population of scores that underlie our sample scores are equivalent, as does the t-test. This means that the ANOVA assumes that the populations that we are comparing via our samples have the same, or at least similar, variance. If the underlying populations have the same or similar variance, we can assume, or at least hope, that the samples of these populations that we are testing will also have the same or similar variance, although there are methods available for handling unequal variances.[1]

ANOVA also assumes that the variables that we are testing with it are normally distributed, and that the underlying population scores that we are testing via samples are independent of one another. As we mentioned in the t-test chapter, this means that the individual data points (observations) in one condition are not related to (are independent of) the observations in the other conditions. To relate this ANOVA assumption to our discussion of samples in Chapter 5, a potential problem with a convenience sample is that it can mean that there is a relationship between members of the sample that violates the assumption of independence. There may be commonalities, for example, between the first-year students who walked past our door, who we conveniently recruited for our experiment in much the same way that a spider recruits flies in its web.

The bad news is that there can be computational problems if we violate the ANOVA's assumptions — for example, if there is differing variance in our experimental conditions, or if our data is not distributed normally (such as by being either negatively or positively skewed, as described in Chapter 2), or if there is a relationship or clustering within our data.

The good news is that the ANOVA is a robust technique that can tolerate some degree of violation of its assumptions, particularly in larger samples, because of the nature of the central limit theorem that was introduced in Chapter 4, although even small amounts of clustering can affect our results. It is still necessary, however, to test for the ANOVA's assumptions, as well as to know what they are, before conducting and interpreting ANOVA analyses. When we run an ANOVA on a computer statistics package, this analysis will generally include a test of the assumption of equivalence of variance, such as the Levene's test. If the result of this test is significant, it means that our assumption of equivalence of variance has been violated and that we should therefore take appropriate action, such as removing outliers.

Underlying principles of calculation

The F-value is calculated on the basis of the following variance ratio:

$$F = \frac{\text{variance between groups}}{\text{variance within groups}}$$

This can also be represented as:

$$F = \frac{\text{treatment effect} + \text{differences due to chance}}{\text{differences due to chance}}$$

Therefore, if there is no treatment effect, $F = 1$.

When we use a computer package to run an ANOVA, the output will provide a summary table that includes an F-value of the differences between our sample means, and also a p-value of the statistical significance associated with our F-value. As was the case with the p-value associated with a t-value, this is the probability of obtaining an overall difference between the groups that was this large, or larger, by chance, if the null hypothesis was actually true. As with the t-test and other inferential statistical measures, a significant statistical effect does not necessarily mean that our result is also clinically meaningful. This distinction is important (although often neglected) and has been mentioned previously. It will be discussed in the context of specific statistics for the health sciences (Chapter 12).

As with t-tests, we use an ANOVA to test the null hypothesis that there is no significant difference between our conditions, and if we obtain a statistically significant difference we reject our null hypothesis. We could perhaps also throw a party if our findings and research budget are sufficiently expansive, but we could do this statistically responsibly only if *the clinical as well as the statistical significance is meaningful*. As with t-values, to achieve a significant F-value means that the variance associated with differences in scores between conditions needs to be considerably larger than the variance associated with differences in scores within conditions (error).

Types of ANOVA: when to use what

ANOVAs come in a range of sizes and varieties. There is an ANOVA that suits many research and clinical needs that involve comparisons of the mean differences between more than two sets of scores. The choice of which ANOVA we should use as our statistical tool begins with the nature of our question and how many variables our question has generated. As with many things, ANOVAs can be conveniently divided into types, and these typologies include one way, two way and so on, and univariate and multivariate. If we have a particularly complex research problem, or if we are just particularly enthusiastic, we can embark on three-way or even four-way ANOVA adventures, but describing these will take us well beyond the safe harbour of this gentle statistical introduction, and these can be seriously difficult to interpret. Which ANOVA we use depends on how many comparisons we would like to make, which will be reflected in how many independent variables we have and also in how many dependent variables we have.

One-way ANOVA

What if our research or other interest involves needing to know the significance of differences between three or more sets of scores? These sets of scores represent levels of a single independent variable, and in this case we can use a one-way ANOVA to analyse our data, because this will allow us to calculate the significance of differences between three or more group means. The one-way ANOVA is so called because it is used in situations where there is only one independent variable, of however many levels. This is also a univariate ANOVA because we apply it to only one dependent variable. We can return to the saffron example that we used in Chapter 7 to illustrate the application of a one-way ANOVA.

In Chapter 7, we used a paired-samples t-test to compare the pre- versus post-treatment cognitive benefits of saffron administered to a group of patients with Alzheimer's disease (AD), using a dependent variable of

TABLE 8.1   GROUP MEANS FOR IMPROVEMENT IN SAFFRON-RELATED
COGNITIVE PERFORMANCE FOR THREE AD SEVERITY GROUPS

Mild AD	Moderate AD	Severe AD
Group mean = 8.2 n = 5	Group mean = 9.2 n = 5	Group mean = 5.7 n = 5

memory score as our measure of cognitive function. We used an independent-samples t-test to compare a saffron treatment with a placebo 'treatment'. What if we are now interested in whether saffron-related cognitive improvement is different for different degrees of AD severity? We can now use a one-way ANOVA to compare cognitive improvement levels of groups of people diagnosed with (1) mild AD, (2) moderate AD and (3) severe AD (Table 8.1). This will allow us to test our null hypothesis that there are no differences in saffron-related cognitive performance improvement between people diagnosed with mild, moderate and severe AD.

Once we have used a computer package to run an ANOVA on our saffron-related cognitive improvement scores, the computer results output will provide us with a summary table that includes an F-value, which is similar to a t-value. This is a measure of the magnitude of the differences between our sample means, calculated for each of the three levels of our independent variable. In this case we obtain an F-value of 11.51, which means that our treatment effect (the variance between our group means) is 11.51 times greater than the error (the variance within our group means). We obtain an associated p-value of <0.05, which our computer has calculated on the basis of our degrees of freedom. In this case, our degrees of freedom for treatment are:

$$k - 1 \,(\text{conditions minus } 1) = 3 - 1 = 2$$

Our degrees of freedom for error are:

$$k(n - 1) = 3(5 - 1) = 12$$

Since our obtained F is higher than our critical level of F, we therefore have a statistically significant result, but not necessarily a clinically significant one, and we will also need to examine our effect size.[2,3] We can therefore reject our null hypothesis that there is no difference between conditions. However, what if we want to know which differences between which group means are responsible for our overall significant result?

Planned and post hoc comparisons

If the overall F is significant, we can use a range of statistical methods to make individual comparisons between our condition means, which may tell us which condition differences are responsible for the overall significant difference between our conditions. A distinction can be made between a priori and post hoc comparisons, which means that we can specify the individual comparisons that we will make before we run our ANOVA (a priori) or after it (post hoc).

There are various types of individual condition comparison methods that we can use, or instruct our computer to use, including the modified least significant difference (LSD) test, the Scheffé test and Tukey's honestly significant difference (HSD) test. These tests are similar to t-tests in that they involve comparisons between just two conditions, and basically reduce the alpha level (our nominated critical level of p, usually 0.05) based on our number of comparisons.

There are important advantages in using individual comparisons within an ANOVA analysis rather than just using a multiple t-test, machine-gun style approach to statistical analysis. These advantages include a reduction in the likelihood that we will make type 1 errors (that we will inappropriately reject our null hypothesis). If we simply ran 100 t-tests to make 100 comparisons between two experimental conditions, we could expect a significant result 5 times out of 100 by chance alone if we are using an alpha of 0.05. Incidentally, the author once observed such an analysis undertaken by a senior researcher at a health-science university department with which he was associated, who should have known better. This singular statistical foray consisted of running 167 t-tests rather than a more appropriate analysis, and it swiftly entered that university department's statistical folklore.

Planned comparisons in action

In our saffron example we can appropriately use planned comparisons to reveal the significance of the differences in memory performance improvement between mild and moderate AD groups, between mild and severe AD groups, between moderate and severe AD groups, and also between any two combined groups and the remaining group. We can instruct our computer package to undertake whichever comparisons interest us, and these vary, as do many of us, in their conservatism. The Scheffé test is particularly conservative, as it is less likely to generate a significant result.

In our one-way ANOVA example, our planned comparisons between group means reveal that there is no statistically significant difference in memory score improvement between mild and moderate AD groups, but that there *is* a significant difference in memory score improvement between both the mild and moderate AD groups and the severe AD group. The severe AD group showed less saffron-related memory improvement than did either of the other two groups. We can therefore state, on the basis of our planned comparisons, that saffron improves cognitive performance less well for people with severe AD than it does for people with mild or moderate AD.

Two-way ANOVA

What if our research or clinical or other interest involves needing to know the significance of differences between two or more levels of one independent variable, and also between two or more levels of a second independent variable? What if we are also interested in whether the relationship between scores on our dependent variable is different across levels of one independent variable from what it is across levels of the other independent variable? This might sound like an extremely unlikely thing for anybody to be interested in, but it is in fact common in at least some areas of health-science research, and how it works may well become clearer via the use of an example.

What if we want to know whether saffron has a different cognitive-function-improving benefit for people diagnosed with AD (across severity levels) for females than it does for males, as well as whether there is a difference in improvement between males and females, and between saffron dose conditions? In this case we can use a two-way ANOVA, which will allow us to calculate the significance of differences between two or more levels of one independent variable, and between two or more levels of a second independent variable. The two-way ANOVA also allows us to calculate whether the differences between levels of one independent variable are greater across levels of our other independent variable. These revelations are known successively as our first main effect, second main effect and interaction effect. The interaction effect is the combined effect of two or more independent variables (predictor variables) on a dependent variable (outcome variable).

The two-way ANOVA is so called because it is used in situations where we have two independent variables, each of however many levels. Again, this is a univariate ANOVA, because we are applying it in situations where we only have one dependent variable. We can add a categorical independent variable (gender) to our Chapter 7 t-test saffron example, which will turn it into an example of a two-way ANOVA, which we can use to test for:

1. the significance of differences between scores pre- and post-saffron treatment on our memory performance DV, which we looked at with a t-test in Chapter 7 — our first main effect.

2. the significance of differences between scores on our memory performance DV between males and females — our second main effect.

3. the significance of the interaction between differences between pre- and post-saffron treatment scores on our memory performance DV and between genders — our interaction effect.

Each of the above three effects will have an associated null hypothesis:

1. that there is no difference in pre- versus post-saffron treatment memory performance

2. that there is no difference in memory performance between males and females

3. that there is no interaction effect — that saffron-related memory-performance improvement is the same for males and for females.

We may not be particularly interested in our second main effect (the potential difference in memory performance between males and females) but we may be particularly interested in examining our interaction effect.

Interaction effects

The interaction effect is often an important aspect of two (and more) way ANOVAs, and we will have a statistically significant one if the effect of one of our independent variables (factor) on our dependent variable is not the same across levels of our other independent variable (factor). For example, an interaction between saffron-related memory score and gender would mean that the effect of the saffron treatment on memory-performance improvement is not the same for males as it is for females. It is far easier to understand an interaction effect if we plot it on a graph than by looking at a table of means.

Remember that it is again vital in our ANOVA analysis that we undertake appropriate preliminary analyses of our data, such as calculating descriptive statistics, plots and graphs, before we embark on more complex analyses.

Repeated-measures ANOVAs

A repeated-measures ANOVA is one in which at least one of its factors consists of a measure that has been given to the same group of participants more than once. Repeated measures are commonly used in the health sciences because they allow researchers and others to control for variability between experimental participants, so that the variance will mostly be due to differences between conditions, rather than differences between individual participants. To put this basic principle another way, if we are testing the same people in more than one condition, we can expect the differences in their scores to be due to differences between experimental conditions, and not between participants.

A two-way repeated-measures ANOVA in action

In our ongoing saffron treatment for AD example, which is now our saffron treatment by gender interaction example, saffron treatment is a within-groups (repeated measures) factor because the same group of people were measured twice — before and after saffron treatment. Gender is a between-groups factor, because it contains different groups of people (male and female). We can use a two-way ANOVA to reveal the significance of differences between sets of means on both of our factors and also for our interaction.

Our two-way ANOVA analysis, with repeated measures on one of our factors, reveals that we have a significant treatment main effect, and also a non-significant gender main effect. More importantly for our research question, our two-way ANOVA reveals that we have a significant

TABLE 8.2 GROUP MEANS FOR PRE- AND POST-SAFFRON TREATMENT MEMORY SCORES BY GENDER

	Pre-treatment	Post-treatment	Overall mean
Females	Group mean = 9.1 $n = 5$	Group mean = 9.3 $n = 5$	9.2
Males	Group mean = 8.9 $n = 5$	Group mean = 9.5 $n = 5$	9.2
Overall mean	9.0	9.4	Grand mean 9.2

Box 8.3 **To repeat or not to repeat?**

The popularity of ANOVA with at least some researchers and others in at least some health sciences has recently declined, and at least some contemporary (informed) statistical thinking considers that repeated-measures ANOVA should be avoided, like plagues and clichés. This increasing reluctance to embrace, or at least use, a familiar and seemingly advantageous technique is in response to several issues, including that repeated measures assume, not always correctly, that there are data for all time points.[4]

New statistical methods, such as advanced hierarchical linear modelling and multilevel modelling, are considered by at least some statistical experts to be more appropriate for use in repeated-measures situations. These techniques are particularly suitable for data with complex patterns of variability — for example, where the variability is contained within embedded structures. An embedded structure is one where there is nested information, such as statistics students in a class, or where there is data that is being measured across a series of time points. The intention of this book, however, is (you may be relieved to be reminded) to provide you with a safe statistical harbour, not a stormy statistical sea, so these advanced statistics will not be discussed any further here. Particularly interested (and courageous) readers are referred to relevant texts such as Howell,[2] Heck and Thomas,[4] and Field.[5]

interaction effect, which means that saffron treatment for AD improves memory performance more for males than it does for females. We can therefore state that saffron significantly improves cognitive performance across males and females (main effect 1) and that it does this more effectively for males that it does for females (interaction).

Even-more-way ANOVAs

If our research or other question involves wanting to know whether there are main-effect differences involving more than two independent variables, and also whether there are interaction effects involving these variables, then we can undertake three-way, four-way and even-more-way ANOVAs. As we add more independent variables, interpreting the results of our ANOVA analyses becomes progressively more complex, and interpreting the interaction effects of three-, four- and even-more-way ANOVAs is not recommended for anyone other than the statistically highly enthusiastic and/or courageous. The basic principle of interpreting interaction effects, however, remains the same in these more computationally challenging analyses as it is for a two-way ANOVA: we are interested in looking at whether the relationship between scores between levels of one or several independent variables differs across levels of subsequent independent variables. We can also conduct multivariate ANOVAs (MANOVAs), where we are interested in comparisons that involve more than one dependent variable, but this is also beyond the scope of this elementary statistical introduction (safe statistical harbour).

Conclusion

ANOVA makes it possible for us to do something that is even more useful than what we can do with a t-test, and that is to test for the significance of differences between more than two sets of means.

This chapter concludes our coverage of statistical tests of differences. In Chapters 9 and 10 we will discuss another major group of inferential statistics — measures of association.

Quick reference summary

- The basic computational principle that underlies ANOVA is the same as the one that underlies t-tests. The measure of difference that it produces — in this case an F-value rather than a t-value — can be seen as a signal (between groups variance) to noise (within groups variance) ratio, or even a wheat-to-chaff ratio.

- Choosing which type of ANOVA to use depends on the nature of our question and how many variables our question has generated.

- ANOVA gives us an overall measure of statistical significance — F. If this is significant, we can use planned comparisons to tell us which of our condition differences are responsible for our overall significant difference.

- A repeated-measures ANOVA is one in which at least one of its factors consists of a measure that has been given to the same group of participants more than once.

References

1. Wilcox RR. *Introduction to Robust Estimation and Hypothesis Testing.* 2nd ed. Boston, MA: Elsevier; 2005.

2. Howell D. *Statistical Methods for Psychology.* 7th ed. Belmont, CA: Duxbury Press; 2010.

3. Cumming G. *Understanding the New Statistics: Effect Sizes, Confidence Intervals, and Meta-analysis.* New York: Routledge; 2012.

4. Heck R, Thomas S. *An Introduction to Multilevel Modeling Techniques.* 2nd ed. New York: Routledge; 2009.

5. Field A. *Discovering Statistics Using SPSS.* 3rd ed. London: Sage; 2009.

Further reading

Jaccard J. *Interaction Effects in Factorial Analysis of Variance.* Thousand Oaks, CA: Sage; 1998.

Maxwell S, Delaney H. *Designing Experiments and Analyzing Data: a Model Comparison Perspective.* 2nd ed. Mahwah, NJ: Erlbaum; 2004.

CHAPTER 9

MEASURES OF ASSOCIATION 1: CORRELATION

Stephen McKenzie and Dean McKenzie

OBJECTIVES

After carefully reading this chapter you will:

- know the underlying principles of correlations
- understand the differences between types of correlation, and when it is appropriate to use which
- have the ability and inclination to do a correlation without the assistance of a computer
- realise the importance of interpreting correlation results carefully
- appreciate the fundamental interconnectedness of all things.

Introduction

What really goes with what? Do birds of a feather really flock together, and if they do, what statistic can give you the precise level of association between bird sociability and flock size? Many of us might think that eating less and living longer always go together, but what is the objective evidence for this? Correlation statistics measure the degree of linear (able to be plotted as a straight line) association or relationship between two variables, and they can answer some really important questions, including those that you might not have even thought of asking yet.

An important principle underlying the correlation statistic is that if two sets of scores are correlated with each other, this may mean that the concepts that underlie them are also related. For example, height and weight are both measures of size and growth, and their characteristics and underlying concepts tend to be associated. Just because measures of two things are associated (such as height and weight), however, it does not necessarily follow that the one has *caused* the other. In other words, there may well be a causal relationship, but we are not able to infer this merely on the basis of a correlational relationship.

Correlations, like news, can be either positive or negative. Height and weight are positively correlated because as one increases, so generally does the other. Temperature and amount of clothing worn are negatively correlated, because as one increases, the other generally decreases. Correlations can be weak or strong, like most relationships. If our first variable (*x*) is sense of humour and our second variable (*y*) is good health, a perfect *positive* correlation between these two variables means that as scores on humour go up, so do scores on good health, and as scores on humour go down, so do scores on good health. This perfect positive linear correlation between two variables is stated as a correlation of 1. A perfect *negative* correlation between sense of humour and good health, however, means that high scores on one of these variables are associated with low scores on the other, so as scores on humour go up, scores on good health go down, or as scores on humour go down, scores on good health go up. A perfect negative linear correlation between two variables is stated as a correlation of −1. If there is no relationship whatsoever between sense of humour and good health, scores on these variables are completely unrelated. A total lack of linear correlation is stated as a correlation of 0.

Many things in nature are related to many other things, which is the nature of nature. Our statistical and life results tend to be related to our efforts, for example, and correlations can tell us just how close these associations are. An important purpose of correlation analyses is to take us farther than a description of levels of association and to suggest testable hypotheses that will help explain *why and how* things are related.

Some correlation commandments

There are three correlation commandments that can affect the limitations of this form of analysis, if we follow them faithfully, which we need to do if our aim is an informed, mutually respectful, consenting, productive long-term successful relationship with statistics, and not just a fling.

1. Correlation does not imply causation.

It is important for you to remember that just because two variables are related, it does not necessarily follow that one has caused the other.[1] A general example of this important correlation principle is that there is a positive correlation between length of skirts and economic gloom, but it is not necessarily true that one has caused the other. It may be that both of these variables are actually influenced by a third variable, such as a relationship between clothing and economic fashions, or the alignment of Pluto with Uranus. Very incidentally Pluto has now been downgraded by the International Astronomical Union from a fully fledged planet to a minor or dwarf planet.[2] Your research design may well have failed to incorporate this ex-planetary causal variable, due to a shortage either of funds or imagination.

A health-science example of the above correlation principle involves the positive correlation that has been found between coffee consumption and lung cancer, but this does not necessarily mean that coffee *causes* lung cancer. A recent analysis undertaken in China of the results of many studies of the relationship between coffee and lung cancer suggests that the relationship is complex, and that there may be an underlying causal factor that is actually associated with both lung cancer and coffee consumption — and that is smoking.[3]

2. Variables in a correlation analysis need to be linearly related.

This correlation commandment can be described more simply as: the relationship between our two variables of interest needs to be a pattern that can be plotted as a straight line. Human height and weight are linearly related because as scores on one of them go up, scores on the other also go up. Two variables that are not linearly, but curvilinearly, related are age and strength. As age goes up so does strength, but only up to a certain point, at which it starts to go down again. (For more about curvilinear relationships, see Box 9.1.)

3. Resist any temptations to use the wrong sort of correlations on categorical or binary data.

This is the third correlation commandment, as this chapter concentrates on measuring associations between two variables that were measured on an interval, ratio or ordinal scale, and we should not use correlations intended for measuring associations between nominal or categorical

Box 9.1 The Yerkes-Dodson law

A very famous health-sciences example of a curvilinear relationship is known as the Yerkes-Dodson law, originally published in 1908 by American psychologist Robert Mearns Yerkes (1876–1956) and his postgraduate student John Dillingham Dodson (1879–1955). Yerkes and Dodson found that as physiological or psychological arousal goes up, so does performance on a particular task, but only up to a certain point, at which it starts to go down again, so the relationship looks like an inverted U-shape.[4]

Although more properly a hypothesis rather than a law, the above relationship has received further empirical support, including from a recent study of nursing and physiotherapy students, which found that academic performance was highest for those with medium levels of academic stress![5] So when sitting down to your next exam, allow yourself enough stress to take it seriously, and read the questions thoroughly, but by all means avoid being too stressed!

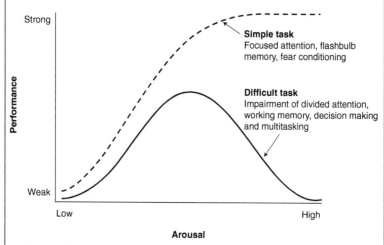

Fig 9.1   The inverted U-shaped curve of the Yerkes-Dodson law

variables on these ratio or interval variables (see Chapter 2 for definitions of these scales). Thus we can appropriately correlate height and weight, skirt length and the Dow Jones Index, the number of official planets in our solar system and the popularity of the International Astronomical Union, and coffee consumption and lung cancer. We cannot, however, appropriately use the methods described in this chapter to correlate eye colour (a nominal or categorical variable) and favourite pizza topping (ditto), although methods for answering such questions are, you may be relieved to know, available.[6]

Correlation preliminaries

It is vital that we start off our correlational relationship with our data by properly acquainting ourselves with it, such as by examining a scatter plot of the relationship between our variables,[7] to ensure that they are in fact linearly related. If they are not linearly related, it may still be possible to proceed, with care, with our correlation — for example, by transforming and therefore reforming our variables back to the linearly straight and narrow. In the case of the Yerkes-Dodson example, we might legitimately suspect a quadratic relationship (in this case represented by an upside down U-shape), with mean academic performance peaking somewhere in the middle of the academic stress curve and being lower for very low stress (as in so calm as to be falling asleep) or very high stress (as in too stressed to do anything but be stressed). We can then transform our academic stress measure by taking the square, which may result in a linear relationship with academic performance.

Some uses and abuses of correlations

We can accurately, and even profitably, see correlational analysis as a useful and objective technique for fulfilling a professional or personal wish to find out how closely associated two or more variables of interest are, and whether this association is statistically significant. If an inferential statistical result is statistically significant, as you may remember from Chapter 6, our chances of getting a result as large as or larger than this one, if the null hypothesis (of no association) is actually true, is 5% or less, with an alpha of 0.05.

To illustrate the above principle with a real health-science example, researchers at the University of Sydney and Concord Hospital found, perhaps surprisingly, that there is only a mild association between eating less and living longer.[8] The authors of this study provided an interesting descriptive statistic that is consistent with the modesty of this correlation. The longest-lived people on our planet — those from the Japanese island of Okinawa — eat about 40% fewer kilojoules than do Americans, and yet live only about 4 years longer. Whether living 4 years longer is a clinically meaningful as well as a mildly statistically significant difference is open to question, and this may depend greatly on what the extra 4 years are spent doing. It may actually be the case, however, that the relationship between kilojoules consumed and years lived is not linear — that there is indeed a strong association between these variables, but only beyond a certain critical age or kilojoule intake.

Another real health-science example of a correlational analysis may assist in your correlational education. Researchers at St Vincent's Hospital in Melbourne, Australia, investigated a possible association between depression and life satisfaction.[9] They were interested in this possible relationship because depression is known to negatively affect prognosis following acute cardiac events such as heart attack and stroke. Increased knowledge of the life factors with which depression is associated may ultimately help to reduce its negative effects and therefore improve post-cardiac events prognoses. This increased knowledge may also reduce a massive worldwide cause of unhappiness and ill health. We will use the example of the relationship between depression and life satisfaction to illustrate the first of two major methods of conducting correlational analyses. Which of these methods we choose depends on some considerations that are described in the following section.

Types of correlations

We can conveniently divide correlations into two main types: those that are appropriate for use with ratio and interval data, and those that are appropriate for use with ordinal data (see Chapter 2 for a reminder of the distinction). Do not worry too much about this distinction, though, because in practice we can actually use the same formula on both types of data, as computers often do.

There are important benefits to learning how to do at least one type of correlation by hand, and therefore not having to rely totally on computers to do them. These benefits are not restricted to such unlikely situations as being stuck on a desert island without a computer or a power point to plug it into, and urgently needing to do a correlational analysis on the level of association between amounts of unknown plants consumed and nausea experienced ('survival statistics'?). The ability to do a correlation by hand, and to at least vaguely understand what you are doing and why, will help to develop your general statistical literacy. The correlation formula given in this chapter is not necessarily the simplest to calculate, but it will be the most helpful illustration of how correlation computations relate to underlying correlation principles.

As briefly stated above, which type of correlation is appropriate for our statistical analysis depends on the nature of our data — the course for our horse. If our data are measured on an interval or ratio scale, which is to say that differences in values are quantitative (horses' best running times around a track, or dollars bet on each horse), then it is appropriate to use a *Pearson product-moment correlation* (for more about Pearson, see Box 9.2). If our data are measured on an ordinal scale, which is to say that our values are ordered (horses coming first, second, third) but the distances between each point may not be equal (difference between first and second

---

Box 9.2 **Setting the statistical scene**

Carl Pearson was born in London in 1857. The very slightly re-badged *Karl* Pearson died in Surrey in 1936. Dr Pearson is popularly said to have officially changed the spelling of his first name in honour of Karl Marx (1818–93), the co-inventor of communism, although there is some doubt about the reason for the name change.[10] As his surname might suggest, Dr Pearson developed the Pearson product-moment correlation coefficient, as well as many other important statistical tests, including the chi-square.

Pearson started his journey to statistically significant superstardom by trying to devise a method to test the theory of evolution. Pearson's inspiration originally came from shrimps (ably assisted by shore crabs). The great evolution researcher and statistician Sir Francis Galton (1822–1911) was Charles Darwin's (1809–82) cousin and the developer of the now famous psychological phrase and concept 'nature versus nurture'. In addition Galton found time to put the identification of fingerprints in criminal investigations onto a sound scientific footing (as it were) and was also an important pioneer of regression (to be described in chapter 10) and correlation.

Other important pioneers of correlation have included Adrien-Marie Legendre (1752–1833), Auguste Bravais (1811–63), Francis Ysidro Edgeworth (1845–1926) and Walter Frank Raphael Weldon (1860–1906).[11] Both regression and correlation were further developed by Pearson, who along with other scientists such as Edgeworth and Weldon was highly inspired by Galton.

---

position may not be anywhere near the difference between second and third), then it is appropriate to use *Spearman's rank-order correlation (Spearman's rho)*, or *Kendall's correlation (Kendall's tau)*. For the sake of simplicity, we will discuss only rho here. Ordinal data include situations where information is lost, such as by reducing horses' complete range of best running times to categories of 'fast', 'average' and 'slow'; or by reducing the number of dollars bet to 'lots', 'some' and 'not much'.

Pearson's product-moment correlation

Underlying principles

The basic principle underlying the Pearson product-moment correlation is that it builds on the notion of covariance, the degree to which two variables vary together, or covary. There are several formulas that can be used (appropriately) to work out this correlation coefficient. The covariance formula that we will use here provides a ratio of the extent to which the two variables vary together (covary) to the extent to which they vary separately. The higher the ratio of the variables varying together, the more the variables are correlated. The numerator (the top part of the correlation formula given below) is actually based on our old friend the variance, which we used in Chapter 3 to calculate standard deviations.

We will translate the covariance correlation formula into English for the compelling reason that this will probably help you understand it.

Calculating a Pearson's correlation

Without further ado, and before you have a chance to escape, we will now get stuck into an example of a Pearson's correlation through which we will guide you step by step. We will use a Pearson's product-moment correlation analysis to answer a real research question — to what extent is depression associated with wellbeing? Although the example is real, the data we employ for the example are not real, they were made up by us — created especially for this chapter. The first thing we need to do before we get our statistical feet wet is establish that we have a linear relationship between our variables, by calculating a scatter plot of their relationship. We will do this for our sample analysis of five hypothetical pairs of depression and wellbeing scores (Fig 9.2).

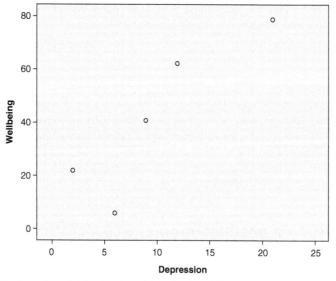

Fig 9.2   **A scatter plot for five hypothetical pairs of depression and wellbeing scores**

The next thing we need to do in order to work out the correlation between our variables, by hand, is to choose a formula. Choosing the right formula might not seem quite as important as choosing the right business or life partner, because all Pearson's correlation formulas lead to home, but, as with most things worth doing, it is best to do this properly. The relatively straightforward 'classical' formula for calculating a Pearson's correlation coefficient starts with calculating the covariance, as described in the top line of the covariance formula lurking below. This formula uses the differences between x scores and the x mean, and the differences between y scores and the y mean, to help us to calculate a ratio of the extent of variables varying together with the extent of variables varying apart. We used aspects of this formula in Chapter 3 to calculate our standard deviations.

The covariance formula for calculating a Pearson's correlation is:[12]

$$r = \frac{\text{cov}_{xy}}{s_x s_y}$$

$$\text{where cov}(xy) = \frac{\sum (x - \bar{x})(y - \bar{y})}{N - 1}$$

Do not worry if this formula looks Greek to you at first fright. This may just be because part of it actually *is* Greek — the capital letter sigma, which is the Greek equivalent of the English capital letter S.

The formula can be translated into English, or something close to it, as:

To calculate the correlation between two variables we firstly work out the top line of the above formula which will give us their covariance (the extent to which they vary together). To do this we subtract the mean of the x *scores from each* x *score, then subtract the mean of the* y *scores from each* y *score, then multiply these two calculated scores by each other.*

Next we add together these products and divide the result by the number of pairs minus one. This gives us the answer to the top line of the overall formula.

To get the answer to the bottom line of the overall formula we multiply the standard deviation of the first variable by the standard deviation of the second variable.

Next we divide the answer to the top line of the overall by our answer to the bottom line of the overall formula. This gives us (at last!) our Pearson's product-moment correlation.

This process can (thankfully) be illustrated as a worked example divided into steps:

1. *Calculate the mean of the x variable and the mean of the y variable.*

In the above example, the *x* variable is depression as measured by the Cardiac Depression Scale (CDS),[13] the *y* variable is wellbeing as measured by the Personal Wellbeing Index (PWI).[14] Incidentally, the CDS was developed by University of Melbourne and Austin Hospital psychiatry and cardiology researcher Professor David Hare and his colleagues. The data presented in the following table are not from the actual study but are simulated (made up by the authors) for the purpose of this example. As will be seen, these data include some (planned) peculiarities, and particularly eagle-eyed readers may wonder about the score of 6 in the PWI column, which is much lower than the other scores.

We have now (finally!) come to the five nominations, that is, to the five pairs of scores:

x	y
CDS	PWI
2	22
21	79
12	62
6	6
9	41
N = 5	

$$\text{Mean } (x) = \frac{2+21+12+6+9}{5}$$
$$= \frac{50}{5}$$
$$= 10$$

$$\text{Mean } (y) = \frac{22+79+62+6+41}{5}$$
$$= \frac{210}{5}$$
$$= 42$$

2. *Subtract the mean of the x scores from each x score, then subtract the mean of the y scores from each y score:*

x − mean (x)	y − mean (y)
2 − 10 = −8	22 − 42 = −20
21 − 10 = 11	79 − 42 = 37
12 − 10 = 2	62 − 42 = 20
6 − 10 = −4	6 − 42 = −36
9 − 10 = −1	41 − 42 = −1
N = 5	

3. *Multiply each of the values obtained in step 2 by each other and then add them together:*

x − mean (x)	y − mean (y)	(x − mean x) × (y − mean y)
−8	−20	160
11	37	407
2	20	40
−4	−36	144
−1	−1	1
		Sum = 752

4. *Divide the answer to step 3 by the number of pairs minus 1:*

$$752 \div 4 = 188$$

$$\text{cov}(xy) = 188$$

We now have the answer to the top line of our overall formula. The size or 'magnitude' of the covariance is related to the spread/scatter/dispersion of the x and y scores around their means, which is to say their standard deviations (see Chapter 4). Therefore a large covariance *may* represent a high association between scores on the depression variable and scores on the wellbeing variable, or it *may not*, depending on the size of the standard deviations of x and y. To remedy this quandary we will now divide $\text{cov}(xy)$ by the answer to the bottom line of our overall formula. To get this answer we will need to multiply the standard deviation of the x (depression) scores by the standard deviation of the y (wellbeing) scores.

Note that we are now breathtakingly close to a final solution, at which point our statistical formula brussels sprouts will instantly transform into our just desserts of ice-cream and jelly, and the blue bird of statistical happiness will sing.

5. *Calculate the SDs as described in Chapter 3, by first squaring the* x *minus* x *mean scores and then the* x *minus* x *means scores that we calculated in step 2, and then adding up the* x *squared values, and then the* y *squared values:*

(x − mean x)²	(y − mean y)²
64	400
121	1369
4	400
16	1296
1	1
Σ = 206	Σ = 3466
N = 5	

6. *Divide each of these summed scores by N − 1 to get the* x *and* y *variances, and then take the square root of each of these and multiply the results:*

$$Sx = \sqrt{(206 \div 4)} = \sqrt{51.50} = 7.18$$
$$Sy = \sqrt{(3466 \div 4)} = \sqrt{866.50} = 29.44$$
$$7.18 \times 29.44 = 211.38$$

7. *Divide the result of steps 1–4 by the result of steps 5–6:*

$$188 \div 211.38 = 0.89$$

Voilà! The correlation between depression and wellbeing as calculated using these five pairs of simulated data is 0.89, which is a strong positive correlation and means in plain language that as depression goes up wellbeing also goes up. In real life (both actual and statistical) such strong correlations are quite rare, so enjoy this rare triumphant moment. Our enjoyment of this result should, however, be moderated by our critical appraisal of its meaning. A strong positive correlation between depression and wellbeing may not be what we expected, or even hypothesised (see Chapter 7), so we can appropriately ask (as US physicist and educator Professor Julius Sumner Miller (1909–87) often did on his long-running Australian TV show) 'Why is it so?'.[15]

A possible answer to our seemingly odd result is that our sample size is very small, and our results might not be equivalent to, or might even be the opposite of, what we might find with a larger sample, although it might also simply be the case that our data has (successfully) simulated 'oddness'.

The researchers in the above study, using real data, actually obtained strong *negative* correlations between these variables (in the order of −0.50), which indicates that as depression goes up, wellbeing goes down, which is what you probably would have expected. You may be realising by now that the process of really getting to know your data — by calculating a statistic on it by hand — can help you to ask questions of it that will lead to a deeply fulfilling relationship.

Squaring our correlation of 0.89 gives us a coefficient of determination, or r square, or an estimate of the amount of variation in our *y* variable (wellbeing) that is explained by the variation in our *x* variable (depression), which is another way of describing the association:

$$r \text{ square} = 0.89 \times 0.89 = 0.79$$

Therefore 79% of the variation in the above wellbeing scores is accounted for by variation in the depression scores (and therefore 21% is accounted for by something we do not yet know about).

Professor Jacob Cohen (1923–98) was a highly influential quantitative psychologist (you may remember him from previous chapters) who suggested that a correlation coefficient ranging from 0.5 up to 1 (or −0.5 to −1) could be classified as a large effect size, although this depends upon the context in which the correlation is being examined.[16] For example, if test–retest reliability (described in Chapter 13) is being assessed, then, arbitrarily but conventionally, correlations need to be 0.70 or higher.

Our correlation of 0.89 therefore suggests that there is a strong relationship between depression and wellbeing, although we need to remember the first correlational commandment — *correlation does not necessarily imply causation*. Wellbeing level may not cause depression, and depression level may not cause wellbeing, even though they are associated. It may actually be the case that both these variables are associated with something we have not measured, such as serotonin levels, which may actually be the true underlying cause of levels of *both* depression and wellbeing. Often in research the answer turns out to be our next question. We also need to remember in interpreting our result that our five observations form only a very small sample and are not accurately representative of anything much at all, apart from the desirability of making life easier for us all than it would have been with a larger sample, and saving calculator batteries.

Interestingly, if we square the actual correlation of 0.50 between *the above two variables that was obtained in the actual study* (that our practice session was based on), we get an *r* square of 0.25. This means that 25% of the variation in the wellbeing scores observed in the actual study are accounted for by the variation in the depression scores, and that therefore 75% of the variation is still a mystery, which is generally the case in actual research involving the measurement of humans. We will return to r square in Chapter 10, on regression.

The next and last question we need to ask of our Pearson's correlation result is: is it statistically significant and what is our estimation of the true or actual population correlation? We can answer this question by calculating the probability that our correlation of 0.89 (or larger) may have arisen by *chance* if the population correlation underlying our sample correlation was actually zero (and not 0.89), meaning that there is no actual underlying relationship between depression and wellbeing. This critical probability value can be calculated using our old and dear friend, the t distribution (see Chapter 8), and by following these steps:

1. *Subtract 2 from the number of pairs (5) to calculate the degrees of freedom = 3.*

2. *Subtract r square (0.79) from 1 = 0.21.*

3. *Divide the result of step 1 (3) by the result of step 2 (0.21) = 14.29.*

4. *Calculate the square root of the result of step 3 = 3.78.*

5. *Multiply the result of step 4 by r* $= 3.78 \times 0.89 = 3.36$

6. *Look up 3.36 in a t table at 3 (number of pairs, minus two) degrees of freedom.*

To be statistically significant at the 0.05 level for 3 degrees of freedom (in this case for 5 observations minus 2), t must be greater than or equal to 3.18, which it is. To be statistically significant at the 0.01 level, t must be greater than or equal to 5.84, which it is not. Therefore our result is statistically significant at the 0.05 level, and we can reject the null hypothesis of zero correlation between depression and wellbeing. We could perhaps also throw a party to celebrate this, if we consider the magnitude of our r square effect size, and our research incidentals budget, to be sufficiently large. In this case we achieved a statistically significant result with a very small sample size, which can be particularly thrilling, but we also need to calmly and soberly consider that if our sample size is sufficiently large, practically any correlation — no matter how miniscule — will not be equal to zero and therefore may be statistically significant. Again, always look at the actual size or practical/clinical importance of your result, and at the nature of the sample on which it was based. Furthermore, as emphasised in Chapter 7 (t-tests), we must wherever possible estimate the value of the population value, in this case correlation, using confidence intervals.

Confidence intervals

It should be noted that, life being what it is, things are not quite as simple as they may appear, and the distribution of the population of all Pearson's r-values does not approximate the normal distribution for small sample sizes. Even when it does approximate normality, for large sample sizes, it is more likely to do so when the true population correlation is zero than for any other value. What all this means is that knowing the rather vague relationship between the actual distribution of population correlations and the normal distribution may not help us all that much if we think the population correlation is actually something other than zero. Therefore, we will need to transform our r-value to normality, using a transformation developed by Sir Ronald Fisher, which is known, perhaps not unreasonably, as Fisher's z transformation or zr transformation. (This should not be confused with the slightly differently spelt Fischer-Z, a British rock band formed at Brunel University in London in the 1970s.) Fisher's z is intended for converting r-values so that they can be referred to a normal distribution, and so make them easier to work with in order to calculate standard errors and confidence intervals.

Once an r-value is transformed to a z-value using Fisher's z transformation, standard errors and confidence intervals can be obtained, which are then 'untransformed' so as to give a confidence interval in terms of our original r. The necessary calculations for this procedure are not all that difficult and can be performed on a calculator, although it would be more usual to use a computer statistical package, such as those described in Chapter 14. The actual formulas, and even more details, are provided in texts such as Chen and Popovich,[6] and Cumming.[17] However, the formulas involve logarithms and, although there is nothing inherently scary about logarithms, for the sake of convenience we will simply obtain the confidence interval 'off-camera' by employing Professor Geoff Cumming's excellent spreadsheet program. This ESCI software, instructions for its use and variations available for two types of operating system can be freely downloaded[18] provided that it is for non-commercial use (and please remember to refer to Professor Cumming's comprehensive textbook[17]).

Using this software (or indeed any relevant statistical packages discussed in Chapter 14) in our correlation example, we obtain a 95% confidence interval of 0.04 to 0.99, which is massively wide. All that can be said, therefore, about this *r-value* is that we can be 95% confident that the true (population) correlation is somewhere between 0.04 and 0.99, which is a little like saying that the proverbial needle is somewhere in the Gobi Desert, or the Pacific Ocean, or the Atlantic Ocean, or the entire planet! What a confidence interval such as this actually means is that if one were to generate an unlimited number of samples of (in this case) 5 observations and calculate the 95% confidence interval for each sample, 95% of these intervals would actually contain the true population value. Although it is sadly true that confidence intervals for Pearson correlations are not computed as often as desirable, they definitely should be computed.

Spearman's rank-order correlation coefficient

Sometimes it is not statistically appropriate to calculate a Pearson's correlation, so in these situations a more robust (that is, less affected by some violations of some statistical assumptions) nonparametric correlation formula that makes fewer assumptions should be used instead. Spearman's rank-order correlation, or *rho*, is perhaps more widely used and easier to calculate than another non-parametric correlation known as Kendall's *tau*, so with apologies to the great British statistician Sir Maurice Kendall (1907–83), we will briefly describe Spearman's *rho*. This test was devised by Charles Spearman (1863–1945), a British psychologist and army officer who resigned from the army in order to do a PhD in experimental psychology in Leipzig, Germany, in 1897 with the great early psychologist Wilhelm Wundt (1832–1920).

Underlying principles

The Spearman correlation builds on the principle that if two sets of ranked scores are perfectly positively linearly correlated there will be no differences between the sum of their ranking orders. If there is a perfect negative linear correlation between the two sets of scores, the total difference of their ranking orders will be the maximum possible. As mentioned above, we should use Spearman's correlation rather than Pearson's correlation if we are using ordinal rather than ratio or interval data. (See Chapter 2 for some useful tips on how to spot the difference.) We may also be able to use Spearman's correlation if we have ratio or interval data containing extreme scores or outliers. By using ranks, Spearman's correlation may be more robust to extreme scores than Pearson's correlation would be.

An invisible formula

There is a formula for calculating Spearman's *rho*, of course, but although it is far simpler than the Pearson's formula there is no need for us to go through it here. Even super-computers in their statistical super-efficiency generally just convert continuously scored variables to ranks, and then run a Pearson's correlation on them. The tests of significance used by computer packages may not be accurate with very small sample sizes (less than 30 or so), however, as they may not allow for the fact that they are actually using ranks[6] although exact tables are available.[19]

More information on Spearman's correlation can be found in Corder and Foreman,[20] while a recent health-science application of the technique is described by Greenop et al, who examined the relationship between pre-stroke personality traits and post-stroke behavioural and psychological symptoms in Australian patients.[21]

Correlation and agreement

It is important to differentiate association in general from a particular type of association known as agreement. For example, two sets of scores given by two raters can have high association but low agreement, as with the scores 1, 2, 3, 4, 5 being highly correlated with the scores 2, 4, 5, 7, 7. The low scores in the first number set are associated with low scores in the second set, and high scores in the first set are associated with high scores in the second set, suggesting a high positive correlation. The agreement does not seem all that high, however, in that the numbers contained in the two sets of scores are never the same across the two sets. This strongly suggests that the two raters never actually agree with each other in terms of their scores.

Measuring the actual agreement between two sets of data (such as observations made by two raters) requires the use of a statistic known as the *intraclass correlation*. The intraclass correlation coefficient is intended to achieve a value of one only if both sets of scores are identical with each other (for example, if both sets of raters assign the same set of scores and the second set of scores is identical to the first). The kappa coefficient is also a measure of agreement, and is intended for measuring agreement on nominal or categorical data (for example, between two raters on medical or psychiatric diagnoses). Indeed intraclass correlation is related to kappa. In practice, the Pearson product-moment and intraclass correlation may give the same results, but it is definitely always best to apply the latter type of correlation when attempting to measure agreement, such as that between two or more sets of scores made by two or more raters. Those who need it can find more information on the intraclass correlation (and kappa coefficient and the specific relationship between them) in Streiner and Norman.[22]

Conclusion

Now that you know what goes with what, and why, you will now be given the thrilling concluding episode of 'Measures of association', parts 1 and 2, in Chapter 10, where you will find out what you need to know, and possibly more, about regression and its allies.

For those who might still be wondering if sense of humour and good health are in fact related, a study reported in the *British Journal of Health Psychology* that was undertaken by researchers at Bond University, on Australia's Gold Coast, investigated this relationship in 504 students, general community members and people with a medical condition.[23] The results of this study suggest that there is indeed a positive association between sense of humour and good health. Remember, however, that this result does not mean that a good sense of humour causes good health, or that good health causes a good sense of humour, it just means that they are linearly associated. Clarification of whether this apparent association actually exists, and what it actually means, may await the inspired research efforts of a particularly inspired reader of *Vital Statistics*.

Quick reference summary

- Correlation is a measure of the association between variables.

- Correlations, like news, can be either positive or negative.

- Correlation does not necessarily imply causation.

- Variables in a correlation analysis need to be linearly related.

- Pearson's product-moment correlation should generally be used to calculate correlations involving ratio and interval data.

- Spearman's rank-order correlation or Kendall's correlation should be used to calculate correlations involving ordinal data and possibly also for ratio and interval data containing extreme scores or outliers.

- It is sadly true that confidence intervals for Pearson (and other) correlations are not computed as often as desirable, but they definitely should be.

- It is important to differentiate association in general from a particular type of association known as agreement.

References

1. Jaccard J, Jacoby J. *Theory Construction and Model-building Skills: a Practical Guide for Social Scientists*. New York: Guilford; 2010.

2. Tyson N, de G. *The Pluto Files: the Rise and Fall of America's Favorite Planet*. New York: Norton; 2009.

3. Tang N, Wu Y, Ma J, et al. Coffee consumption and risk of lung cancer: a meta-analysis. *Lung Cancer*. 2010;67(1):17-22.

4. Yerkes RM, Dodson JD. The relationship of strength of stimulus to rapidity of habit-formation. *Journal of Comparative Neurology*. 1908;18:459-482.

5. Sarid O, Anson O, Yaari A, et al. Academic stress, immunological reaction, and academic performance among students of nursing and physiotherapy. *Research in Nursing & Health*. 2004;27:370-377.

6. Chen PY, Popovich PM. *Correlation: Parametric and Nonparametric Measures*. Thousand Oaks, CA: Sage; 2002.

7. Wainer H. *Graphic Discovery: a Trout in the Milk and Other Visual Adventures*. Princeton, NJ: Princeton University Press; 2005.

8. Everitt AV, Le Couteur DG. Life extension by calorie restriction in humans. *Annals of the New York Academy of Sciences*. 2007;1114:428-433.

9. Page KN, Davidson P, Edward KL, et al. Recovering from an acute cardiac event — the relationship between depression and life satisfaction. *Journal of Clinical Nursing*. 2010;19(5-6): 736-743.

10. Hald A. *A History of Mathematical Statistics from 1750 to 1930*. New York: Wiley; 1998.

11. Heyde CC, Seneta E. *Statisticians of the Centuries*. New York: Springer; 2001.

12. Howell D. *Statistical Methods for Psychology*. 7th ed. Belmont, CA: Duxbury Press; 2010.

13. Hare DL, Davis CR. Cardiac depression scale: validation of a new depression scale for cardiac patients. *Journal of Psychosomatic Research.* 1996;40:379-386.

14. International Wellbeing Group. *Personal Wellbeing Index.* 4th ed. Melbourne: Australian Centre on Quality of Life, Deakin University; 2006. Available online at <http://www.deakin.edu.au/research/acqol/instruments/wellbeing-index/index.php>>. Accessed 23 September 2012.

15. ABC Science. *Why is it so?* Available online at <http://www.abc.net.au/science/features/whyisitso/>>. Accessed 23 September 2012.

16. Cohen J. *Statistical Power Analysis for the Behavioral Sciences.* 2nd ed. Hillsdale, NJ: Erlbaum; 1988.

17. Cumming G. *Understanding the New Statistics: Effect Sizes, Confidence Intervals, and Meta-analysis.* New York: Routledge; 2012.

18. La Trobe University, School of Psychological Science. *The New Statistics: Estimation for Better Research.* Available online at <http://www.latrobe.edu.au/psy/research/projects/esci>>. Accessed 23 September 2012.

19. Siegel S, Castellan NJ. *Nonparametric Statistics for the Behavioral Sciences.* 2nd ed. New York: McGraw-Hill; 1988.

20. Corder GW, Foreman DI. *Nonparametric Statistics for Non-Statisticians: a Step-by-Step Approach.* Hoboken, NJ: Wiley; 2009.

21. Greenop KR, Almeida OP, Hankey GJ, et al. Premorbid personality traits are associated with post-stroke behavioral and psychological symptoms: a three-month follow-up study in Perth, Western Australia. *International Psychogeriatrics.* 2009;21:1063-1071.

22. Streiner DL, Norman GR. *Health Measurement Scales: a Practical Guide to their Development and Use.* 4th ed. New York: Oxford University Press; 2008.

23. Boyle GJ, Joss-Reid JM. Relationship of humour to health: a psychometric investigation. *British Journal of Health Psychology.* 2004;9:51-66.

CHAPTER 10

MEASURES OF ASSOCIATION 2: REGRESSION

Dean McKenzie and Stephen McKenzie

OBJECTIVES

After carefully reading this chapter you will:

- understand the principles underlying principles of regression

- recognise the differences between regression and correlation, and when it is appropriate to use each

- recognise the differences between types of regression, and when it is appropriate to use each

- realise the importance of interpreting regression results carefully

- appreciate that statistical and life opportunities increase when we understand our passage from the known to the unknown.

Introduction

Regression is related to correlation in that it allows us to calculate the extent of linear relationships between variables. Regression differs from correlation in that it gives us a formula, known as a regression equation, that allows us to describe a predictive relationship between variables, even though this 'prediction' can be of concurrent variables, such as depression and physical health levels, measured at the same point in time. Prediction is used here in the sense that it is often used in introductory statistics books: that of estimating values of y from x, even if both are measured at the same time. (More technically, for example in the scientific literature, prediction generally means estimating future values, so please note that we are using it in the widest, estimation, sense here.) Based on the characteristics of our x variable, such as physical health level, what is our best guess of the characteristics of our y variable, such as depression level? This could be stated more formally as: 'For a given value of x, what is the average value of y?' Regression can be seen as a statistical process of predicting, or estimating, the unknown based on the known. The more strongly the characteristics of variables are related, the more accurately we can predict or estimate characteristics of one variable based on knowing the characteristics of one or more other variables.

Odds ratios and relative risks are also very commonly used in a wide range of health sciences. These also relate to prediction in the sense that they can give us vital information about the odds or risk of y, where y can be a disease or consequence of a disease, given our knowledge of a person's scores on a range of relevant associated factors — our x variables. Odds ratios and relative risks will be covered in Chapter 12, and linear regression (for dimensional dependent variables such as scores on a measure of health-related quality of life) will be covered in this chapter. We will also briefly discuss binary logistic regression (for binary dependent variables such as presence or absence of major depression). In doing this we will expand on the principles and calculations to which we introduced you in earlier chapters.

Regression — an overarching system

Jacob Cohen (1923–1998) was a US quantitative psychologist who substantially helped to develop the concepts of effect size and statistical power, which we cover in other chapters. Cohen gave the information science world the Cohen's kappa measure of chance-corrected agreement r and the Cohen's d measure of effect size. He also gave the information science world a classic methodological paper in 1968, in which he demonstrated that analysis of variance (ANOVA) and related statistical techniques such as multiple regression are actually fundamentally identical in theory (in terms of the 'general linear model'), but that in practice multiple regression can readily allow analyses that would be difficult to perform using

Box 10.1 **Setting the statistical scene**

We introduced you to some of the key players in the development of regression in Chapter 9 — Galton and Pearson — but here is some specific contextual information about regression that might help you understand it by placing it in a broader perspective.

Sir Francis Galton (1822–1911) was a multifaceted scientific genius who helped to develop the concept of regression, as well as the concepts of the normal distribution and correlation, with the latter further developed by Karl Pearson. Galton built upon the work of earlier scientists such as Adrien-Marie Legendre (1752–1833) and Carl Friedrich Gauss (1777–1855).[1]

Perhaps interestingly and even famously, Galton observed and described a principle that he called regression towards mediocrity but which is now referred to as regression towards the mean, or regression to the mean, or statistical regression, which we shall discuss in more detail in Box 10.2. But first we set the immediate statistical scene by looking at a landmark paper in the health sciences, concerned with regression — or rather multiple linear regression — as a 'general data-analytic system'.

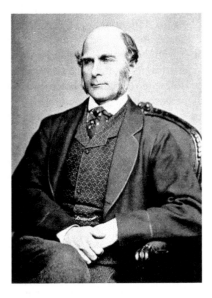

Fig 10.1   **Sir Francis Galton**

ANOVA.[2] The relationship between ANOVA and multiple regression was already well known by statisticians, but may have been less familiar to general health-science researchers, clinicians and other practitioners.

There has been a growing tendency for health scientists and other users and abusers of statistical tests to conduct multiple linear regression rather than ANOVA analyses, although ANOVA is still widely used. It needs to be kept in mind, however, that ANOVA and regression are not 'competitors', and that whatever ANOVA can do, regression can also do, and more. In practice, it may well be simpler to perform a one-way ANOVA using an ANOVA procedure in a statistics package — such as those that will be outlined in Chapter 14 (which will also readily provide post-hoc multiple comparison tests) — than to perform the same analysis using a multiple regression procedure. For more complex designs, however, where you may wish to adjust or statistically control for the potential effects of several variables (as discussed later in this chapter), employing a multiple regression procedure would allow greater flexibility.[3]

An underlying principle of regression

To keep things simple, we shall begin with simple linear regression, which is used to try to predict or estimate the values of a dependent variable, such as health-related quality of life, from a single predictor or independent variable, such as weekly income in dollars or other currency. The basic principle underlying statistical regression methods is simply that our best guess about the characteristics of one variable (in this case) will be based on our knowledge of characteristics of a single related variable (in this case). The more closely our variables are related, the better our guess. Simple linear regression is similar to correlation in that it tests for the relationship between variables, but it differs from correlation in terms of how it conceptualises this relationship. Correlation is fundamentally a test of association, whereas regression is fundamentally concerned with prediction, although not necessarily with predicting scores in the future (as it can be, and often is, used with cross-sectional data, measured at a single point in time).

Regression versus correlation

The fundamental difference between regression and correlation can be seen as being a difference in style rather than of substance. Whether we use correlation or regression or both depends on whether the nature of the relationship or relationships that we are interested in calculating is more naturally conceptualised as prediction/explanation or associations. Sometimes the choice between whether to conduct a correlation or a regression will not be clear cut and will depend mainly on which type of analysis better suits our research question; often we may perform both types of analysis. If we instruct a computer package to conduct a simple linear regression analysis, we will generally get a 'free' Pearson product-moment correlation r value thrown in as part of the computational deal, and it is generally appropriate to calculate both correlations and regressions. There can be an art to statistical science, just as there can be a science to statistical art.

The basic principle underlying linear regression, and how this differs from the basic principle underlying correlation, can be illustrated by a classic example of correlation — the linear relationship between height and weight. Statistical learners are often traditionally introduced to the concept of association via the phenomenon that as height goes up weight also tends to go up — a positive correlation. This is similar to the example traditionally used to introduce statistical learners to probability — that if we throw a coin in the air the chances of it coming down either heads or tails are 0.5. The chances of a fair coin landing heads or tails will indeed be 0.5, no matter how intricate the research hypothesis that inspired the throw, and human heights are indeed generally linearly and positively correlated with weights, no matter how high or how heavy.

What the above universal truths may lack in surprise or creative value they gain in simplicity — the basic believability that makes good bedtime stories and statistical explanations. In this spirit of appropriate respect for tradition, statistical or otherwise, we will begin our illustration of regression with an adaptation of the height and weight example given in Chapter 9.

Greater weights are generally associated with greater heights, and correlations can reveal this positive relationship. Remember that we can also have negative relationships (although not generally for height and weight!), in which as scores on one variable go up, scores on the other go down (such as the relationship between depression and physical health). Another way of looking at a relationship between two sets of scores is: 'To what extent can we predict or estimate weight values based on our knowledge of height values?'; or, 'To what extent can we predict or estimate height values based on our knowledge of weight values?' If we know the extent of the relationship between our variables of interest, we can answer these questions. If two variables are perfectly associated, then knowledge of the characteristics of one variable will give us perfect knowledge of the characteristics of the other variable. This means that we can use our knowledge about one variable to help us predict the characteristics of another variable. If there is a total linear association between values on two variables, then (a) as scores on one of them go up or down so will scores on the other (a perfect positive correlation); or (b) as scores on one of them go up, scores on the other go down, or vice versa (a perfect negative correlation). In linear regression terms, if two variables are perfectly positively or negatively correlated with each other, this means that we can predict or estimate values on one based on our knowledge of values of the other with perfect accuracy.

Regression in the health sciences

Regression is often used in the health sciences to explain or estimate the values of variables in cross-sectional studies. For example, we may conduct a survey in which we measure levels of health-related quality of life, and then examine the relationship between that dependent or target or criterion variable, and our independent or explanatory or 'predictor' variable of weekly income. A simple linear regression will give us an r-squared value (the amount of variation in health-related quality of life that is explained or accounted for by levels of income, assuming the two are linearly related), as well as a regression equation that we could use to answer the question, 'How much will average levels of health-related quality of life increase with each dollar increase in weekly income'?

In reality, many other variables apart from income may have bearing on health-related quality of life. Physical and psychological health — including pain levels — are other variables that may well have an effect on health-related quality of life. An extension of simple linear regression, known as multiple linear regression, allows us to statistically 'adjust for' or 'control for' or 'take into account' the effects of physical and psychological health in estimating the relationship between weekly income and health-related quality of life, for example. It must be emphasised however, that correlation does not necessarily imply causation in the case of regression, any more than it does for correlation, particularly in the case of cross-sectional data.

Regression assumptions

As with all statistical techniques, simple and multiple linear regression make assumptions about our data that we should check before summoning their powers, such as by running preliminary analyses, including scatterplots. As with many statistical techniques, regression assumes that our data is normally distributed in that our *residuals* are normally distributed. This means that the differences (residuals) between our observed or actual dependent variable values and the dependent variable values that we predicted or estimated on the basis of our regression equation are normally distributed. Linear regression makes various other assumptions about our data, including that the variance of the residuals around our predicted or estimated scores is equivalent for all our predicted scores.[3,4] Perhaps not surprisingly, linear regression assumes that the relationship between our dependent and independent variable(s) is linear, or can be transformed to linearity by squaring or cubing the relevant independent variable (in the case of curvilinear — U-shaped or inverted U-shaped — relationships, for example).

To make statistical inferences regarding populations, linear regression assumes that for any given value of x (or multiple xs in the case of multiple linear regression), y is normally distributed, which is equivalent to assuming that the residuals are normally distributed. As with many other statistical techniques, linear regression results can be unduly influenced by the presence of extreme scores, or outliers, and the non-independence of observations. Examples of non-independent observations include people tested more than once, or people from the same street being tested, or the existence of any other systematic testing characteristic that makes the data more correlated than desirable in terms of regression assumptions. It might be reassuring for you to know that methods of regression are available that are resistant or robust to the effects of outliers and can deal with non-independent observations and non-linear relationships not able to be transformed to normality.[3,5]

Types of regression

You may have realised by now that many things, including statistical tests, can be appropriately and usefully divided into types. This subdivisional opportunity is also offered by regression, and as with many things that can be divided into types this subdivision is best done on the basis of intended usage. Which type of regression we should use will logically be determined by what we intend to use it for. *Simple linear regression* involves the calculation of the predictive relationship between one predictor or explanatory or independent variable (known as the x variable) and one criterion variable (known as the y variable). This technique can be used in situations where we are interested only in the relationship between any single predictor variable and any single criterion variable. As described above, *multiple regression* extends this concept to situations where we have more than one x variable.

There are other varieties of regression, such as several flavours of *logistic regression*, which are intended for a binary or categorical y variable (or even for an ordinal y variable) and one or more dimensional or categorical x variables. We will briefly describe other forms of regression later in this chapter (see 'Not-quite-so-simple regression'), so that you will not be unduly perturbed if you should unexpectedly come across one of them in the (research) wild, or at least the need to understand and therefore tame one. The basic principles and calculation characteristics of simple linear regression also apply to other forms of regression, however, and it is much easier to calculate a simple linear regression by hand than it is to calculate other types of regression.

Simple linear regression

We introduced you to the scatterplot in Chapter 9, which illustrated the pattern of relationship between two variables (x and y) in the context of a correlation analysis. With the help of a computer we can add a regression line to our scatterplot. The regression line can be seen as a summary of the relationship between two variables, assuming a linear relationship and that the regression line, or 'line of best fit', actually fits our data. By observing a scatterplot of our actual scores and a regression line of predicted scores based on the regression equation or model, we can see how well the model fits reality (or how well reality fits the model!).

In a simple linear regression analysis, our two variables are described as our independent or explanatory predictor variable (x) and our dependent or target or criterion variable (y), which must be dimensional. If we have one or more categorical xs, we could analyse them using multiple linear regression, using 'dummy' variables, for example.[3,4] We can use the regression line to estimate observed values (scores) on our y variable, based on our observed values (scores) on our x variable. These estimations can be made for any value of y based on any value of x, although it is best not to extrapolate beyond the limits of our data.

If the tallest person in our height sample is 1.85 metres tall, it is best not to work out the weight of someone who is 2.2 metres tall, as we do not actually have valid data with which to make this inference. It should be borne in mind, incidentally, that in the case of predicting weights (y variable) from heights (x variable), our y variable is usually influenced by things other than our x variable. Weight, for example is also affected by age, in that as we grow older, we get taller, and weigh more. Weight is also affected by muscle size and waist size (perhaps even ear size), as well as by height. This is where multiple linear regression can be useful, in that it can tell us what the relationship is between height and weight when we adjust or statistically control for the effects of other variables by holding them constant. We will describe multiple linear regression in more detail below.

Simple linear regression in the health sciences

Medical prognosis provides a good health-science example of naturally and usefully measuring the relationships between variables in a predictive manner, where the prediction is actually of something that will occur in the future. To make an accurate prognosis (prediction), we need to know the extent of the relationship between our potentially predictive variables and our outcome variable (our target or criterion variable). Potentially predictive variables could include severity of illness symptoms, age, marital status, treatment compliance and genetic predisposition. Our criterion variable could be total healthcare cost. We could use a simple linear regression to predict a person's likely total healthcare cost (y variable value), based on knowing their score on a single predictor variable such as severity of illness (x variable). In reality, we would usually prefer to take the possible effects of other variables such as severity of illness, age and marital status into account, and hence we would use multiple linear regression.

Remember that in regression we are often interested in 'predicting' or estimating concurrent events based on our knowledge of other concurrent events, which in the case of this example would mean that we already have the total healthcare cost data that we are 'predicting' or estimating. In this situation, we may be more interested in looking at the effects of one variable, holding other variables constant, or at how much of the variation in y we can explain using x, which is measured by the square of the multiple correlation R, or R^2. In situations where we are interested in predicting total healthcare cost on the basis of more than one predictor variable, and also in determining the relationships between these predictor variables, we would need to use more complex forms of regression, such as multiple linear regression.

As already mentioned, we can conduct a simple linear regression analysis in situations similar to those where we might also consider conducting a correlation analysis (which is closely related to regression). We will therefore use the same example to illustrate the workings of a regression that we used for correlation in Chapter 9, one that involved calculating the level of association between an x variable (scores on the Cardiac Depression Scale, CDS) and scores on a y variable (Personal Wellness Index, PWI) on simulated (invented) data. In that situation, our research interest was to find out to what extent scores on these two variables were linearly associated. What if our research interest is now in how well we can estimate scores on the PWI based on our knowledge of scores on the CDS, or in knowing by how much PWI scores will change with every unit increase on CDS? In this case we could appropriately undertake a simple linear regression analysis rather than, or as well as, a correlation analysis.

Calculating y for particular values of x

The simple linear regression equation allows us to calculate particular predicted or estimated values of our y variable, based on our knowledge of particular x values. The more closely our x and y variables are related, the more accurate our prediction of y values will be. In the example of predicting likely healthcare costs on the basis of severity of illness symptoms, our x (predictor) variable is the severity of illness symptoms, and our y (criterion) variable is total healthcare costs. In the example of predicting PWI scores on the basis of CDS scores, our x (predictor or explanatory) variable is CDS score and our y (criterion) variable is PWI score.

The regression line shows us the relationship between our x and y variables, assuming this relationship is linear, otherwise if we are using linear regression we would need to transform the non linear variables, if it is in fact possible and practical to do so We use the linear regression equation to calculate the regression line, and this can be seen as a line of best fit between scores on these variables. The regression line can be calculated using the formula:

$$\hat{y} = bx + a$$

This can be described in English, or something reasonably close to it as:

y-hat (the predicted value of our y variable) equals the slope of our (x, y) regression line multiplied by the actual value of our x variable plus the intercept of our regression line.

To obtain values for the slope and the intercept of our regression line we need to do some calculations, or instruct a friendly (usually) computer statistical package such as those outlined in Chapter 14 to do these calculations for us. We will now take you through a simple linear regression version of our earlier correlation example, step by step, which involves calculating a particular PWI score on the basis of a particular CDS score. In our correlation example we used the covariance formula to calculate a Pearson's product-moment correlation coefficient of the relationship between these variables, which is a similar formula to the one for calculating a regression equation.

1. *We calculate the slope of our regression line.*

The slope of our regression line shows us how much difference there is in our predicted *y* variable score (PWI) corresponding to one unit difference in our mean *x* variable score (CDS), assuming a linear relationship (or a curvilinear relationship that has been transformed to linearity, if this is in fact possible). Slopes may be positive, negative or even zero (no association between the *x* and *y* variables). In this example, a slope of 0.5 would mean that as scores on CDS increase by one unit, we would also expect predicted scores on PWI to increase (as the slope is positive) by 0.5. We calculate the slope of our regression line by dividing the covariance by the variance of our *x* variable. We calculated the covariance in Chapter 9 for correlation, and we can do this again here within the regression slope formula:

$$b = \frac{cov\,xy}{S^2x}$$

This can be described in words as:

The slope of the regression line equals the covariance of the x and y variables, divided by the variance of the x variable.

In Chapter 9 we obtained a covariance for the relationship between our *x* variable (CDS) and our *y* variable (PWI) of 188 ($N = 5$). We can now insert this value into the top line of our worked equation, in much the same way as TV chefs insert some previously parboiled potatoes into their currently demonstrated display dish. In this case we are working towards creating a complete regression equation rather than a soufflé surprise, but the underlying principles are broadly equivalent. Our standard deviation for *x* was calculated in the correlation example as 7.18, which means that the variance of *x* (CDS) is 7.18^2 (or actually $(7.176)^2 = 51.5$. Our slope is therefore:

$$\frac{188}{51.5} = 3.65$$

This means that for every unit of increase in our x variable score (CDS) we can expect a mean increase of 3.65 in our predicted y variable score (PWI).

> 2. *We calculate the intercept of our regression line.*

The intercept of our regression line reveals what the predicted or estimated value of our y variable (PWI) score will be when the value of our x variable (CDS) score is zero. In many research situations the calculation of the intercept is necessary merely for mathematical reasons and is conceptually meaningless, because in many cases an x score of 0 is meaningless (for example, zero height or weight). As in many situations in life and its statistics, however, we sometimes need to do something just because it needs to be done, rather than for any particular reason. The formula for calculating the intercept is:

$$a = \overline{y} - b\overline{x}$$

This can be described in English as:

> *The intercept of the regression line equals the mean of the y variable minus (the slope multiplied by the mean of the x variable).*

We can then insert into this formula the slope value that we calculated above and the following values (ingredients) that we calculated in Chapter 10:

$$a = 42 - (3.65 \times 10)$$
$$a = 5.5$$

> 3. *We calculate the regression equation.*

We can now insert our slope and intercept values into our regression equation, which gives us:

$$\hat{y} = 3.65 \text{ (slope, or the multiplier of each } x \text{ value)}$$
$$+ 5.5 \text{ (intercept value)}$$

The regression equation gives us particular predicted values of y based on particular values of x, which we can now plot as a regression line on our scatterplot of x and y values. We can start by plotting predicted y values for a low x value and for a high x value. If our x values range from 0 to 10, for example, we can calculate these two y values by inserting 0 and 10 into our formula, which will give us:

$$\hat{y} = 3.65\,(0) + 5.5, \text{ where } x = 0$$

and

$$\hat{y} = 3.65\,(10) + 5.5, \text{ where } x = 10$$

We simply substitute each x value into the regression equation and then plot the results on a graph (Fig 10.2), although in reality, computer statistical packages make it easier (see Chapter 14).

Now that we have calculated a regression line, we can predict y scores for each value of x, and obtain various statistical significance levels. As with many other statistical analyses, it is also useful to calculate confidence intervals — in this case, values can be obtained for the slope, intercept and predicted value of y. We will not take you through regression confidence interval or p-value calculations, because we provided both of these for the r-value in the correlations chapter.

To really get to know regression, you would also have to know about other things, such as the sum of squares (regression) and the sum of

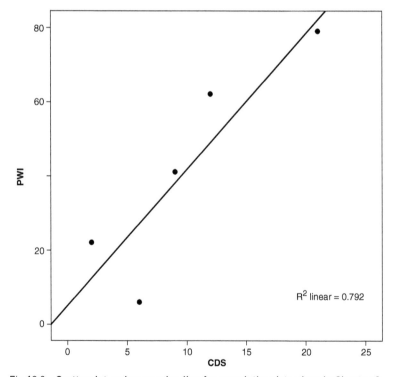

Fig 10.2 Scatterplot and regression line for correlation data given in Chapter 9, assuming a linear relationship

squares (error) — also known as the sum of squares (residual) — which are the same overall concepts as the sum of squares (between groups) and sum of squares (within groups) in ANOVA. However, rather than further burdening you with more formulas, we will simply inform (warn?) you here about the existence of such concepts.[3,4]

Not-quite-so-simple regression

Multiple linear regression

What if we are interested in determining how well more than one predictor variable can predict scores on a criterion variable? In the first regression example above we had the following possible predictor variables: illness symptoms; other possibly influential variables such as age, marital status, treatment compliance and genetic pre-dispositions; and an outcome variable (our target or criterion variable) of total healthcare cost. Multiple regression allows us to enter all the possible predictor or explanatory variables (or at least those it makes make good theoretical sense to include) into a regression equation. This is better than including every possible variable, whether or not there is a good theoretical reason for including them. This process will allow a measure of prediction of our criterion variable to be calculated for all the predictor variables at once, and will allow us to look at the effect of our variable of interest (such as illness symptoms) while holding other variables such as age constant.

The measure of how well a dependent variable can be predicted in multiple linear regression is R^2, which is the measure of how much variance in the y variable is accounted for by the x variables and is obtained by squaring the multiple correlation coefficient R. This is also the case in simple linear regression, where R^2 is the measure of how much variation in the y variable is accounted for by variation in the x variable. We could include all five possible predictor variables mentioned in the above example in a multiple regression analysis and obtain a result such as an R^2 of 0.32. We would certainly not include five predictors if we had only five observations, however, because if the number of predictors equals the number of observations in standard multiple linear regression,[6] R will be 1.0, yet totally meaningless!

An R^2 of 0.32 means that these five predictor variables together explain 32% of the variance in our criterion variable, total healthcare cost. A multiple regression analysis typically also gives us a p-value of the statistical significance and a confidence interval of the relationship between each predictor variable and the dependent variable. Again we need to be careful not to confuse a result that is statistically significant with a result that is clinically meaningful. If we have a large enough sample size, even a clinically trivial result such as an R^2 of 0.03 can be statistically significant. This result would mean that 3% of the variance in our criterion variable has been explained by our predictor variables, which also means that that 97% of our criterion variance is unexplained — it is caused by, or associated with, something that we have not included in our analysis, such as a predictor that we have not included, or a non-linear effect of a predictor that we *have* included but assumed had a linear effect.

Stepwise multiple regression

When there are many potential predictor variables, a smaller set of 'key' variables may be useful in predicting or explaining a target variable that particularly interests us. Such winnowing down of potential variables is often done of the basis of our theoretical and practical experience. Sometimes, however, health-science (and other) researchers may at the very least supplement such knowledge and experience by using computer-based statistical techniques, including one known as *stepwise multiple regression.* This technique has been used (and unfortunately often misused) since the late 1950s.[7]

In theory, but not always in practice, stepwise multiple regression may help us to find out which of our predictor variables are best at predicting or estimating scores on a criterion variable, such as total healthcare cost. Stepwise multiple regression can either be forward-entry regression (where the best single predictor variable among predictor variable candidates is successively selected at each stage or step of the equation-building process) or backward elimination (where the worst single predictor variable candidate is successively eliminated at each stage or step). Stepwise multiple regression can also attempt to combine both these approaches — for example, by at each step either adding the best single predictor or deleting the worst single predictor.[4]

In theory, stepwise multiple regression scenarios may resemble real-life situations where we keep picking the best of something or where we keep eliminating the worst of something — for example, when we are choosing wines or friends, or otherwise making inferences about populations based on sample characteristics without formally doing statistics. In practice, however, stepwise regression is more like trying to choose a champion team based on choosing champion individual players, in that the automated stepwise regression process looks at only one variable at a time, rather than using more of a 'look ahead' or 'looking at combinations' strategy such as choosing a team based on how well players, or variables, perform together.[8]

Stepwise regression may miss variables that actually only perform well in combination; when two variables are about equally good this technique can choose only one of them and so may give the impression that one is better than the other. In other words, stepwise regression may merely select variables on the basis of chance relationships, while the tests of statistical significance that are normally provided in stepwise regression procedures usually do not take all such 'picking and choosing' into account. Just because a predictor variable is not chosen in a stepwise multiple regression, it does not necessarily mean that it is not a good predictor of our criterion variable.[3,9]

Stepwise multiple regression in the health sciences

Stepwise multiple regression (and also stepwise logistic regression) are often used in health-science applications, for example to help identify potential key predictors of the severity of depression in an Australian data set.[10] However, for the reasons discussed above (for example, possibly choosing 'noise' variables or missing 'signal' variables) if stepwise methods are used at all, they should be used extremely cautiously.

Stepwise regression may arguably be best employed in pioneering or hypothesis-generating research,[3] where relationships discovered can be further tested by validating them on other data sets. New methods of validating stepwise regression models, using computer-intensive methods such as the bootstrap described in Chapter 14, are gradually becoming available,[11,12] but unfortunately it takes time for such methods to be accessible to the average user. These new bootstrap methods have not yet quite solved the problem of picking the most important variables (separating signal from noise),[13] but will help to generate regression models or equations that provide good performance when generalised to data sets not used to create the models in the first place.[11] Variable selection, as well as model validation, are exciting ongoing areas of statistical research. In the meantime, caution should always be exercised with any automated procedure, including stepwise regression, and judgment should always be carefully applied.

Some applications of multiple linear regression to Australian data can be found in references 11, 14, 15 and 16.

Logistic regression

Binary logistic regression is another form of regression commonly used in the health sciences and allows us to predict or examine binary outcomes. Polytomous logistic regression is intended for use with categorical outcome variables with three or more values, such as medical diagnosis or ethnicity, and ordinal logistic regression is intended for use with outcomes measured on an ordinal scale, such as age or income ranges.[17]

We may be interested, for example, in examining the relationship between a binary outcome, such as the presence or absence of major depression, and one or more predictor or explanatory variables. Disease is often measured on a binary scale (condition present or absent), although such treatment of information can be non-optimal (as mentioned in Chapter 2), especially if (for some odd reason) we reduce multiple scores on a multiple-item scale effectively to just two scores (such as reducing the 30-item mini-mental status examination to dementia present and dementia absent).

Logistic regression in the health sciences

In a recently published health-sciences example of logistic regression in action, researchers examined the relationship between test items measuring demoralisation (feelings of helplessness and or hopelessness) and anhedonia (loss of interest or pleasure in activities)[18] and the presence or absence of major depression in Australian medically ill hospital patients.[19] As the y or dependent variable (major depression) was binary, binary logistic regression was employed. This technique allowed the researchers to examine the relationship between each item, such as feelings of pessimism and feelings of worthlessness, and the presence or absence of major depression, while adjusting for the presence or absence of all the other items.

Logistic regression generally provides information in the form of odds ratios (for example, the probability of major depression increases when particular items, such as pessimism, are present). For other examples of logistic regression applied to Australian data, see the studies described in references 20–23. For more information on both linear and logistic regression, see Further Reading, as well as references 3, 4 and 17.

Regression towards the mean

Now that you are clear (hopefully!) on the meaning of regression in the sense of a statistical technique to predict or estimate or explain something, let us return to something that is perhaps even more interesting — regression towards the mean. The example that Galton used to illustrate the phenomenon of regression *towards mediocrity* or *towards the mean* is that short parents tend to have children who are taller than they are, and tall parents tend to have children who are shorter than they are. Galton was particularly interested in the latter, hence his concept of regression towards mediocrity, using 'regress' in the sense of the Latin *regressus*, meaning 'a return'.[24] Regression in this sense is an interesting characteristic of nature and relates to the normal distribution, in that phenomena tend to occur most frequently around their average value.

Regression towards the mean has been interpreted by people of limited statistical literacy as a demonstration of a cosmic compensatory force, but it is actually more to do with the simple fact that extremes are less likely to be followed by other extremes (see Box 10.2). If there really were a cosmic compensatory mechanism at play, the life players who believe in it (such as the gamblers who think that a roulette wheel spin 'has to' come up red to 'compensate' for a series of black results) would be correct. Perhaps unfortunately, they rarely are. Statistical procedures tend to relate to and be inspired by naturally occurring phenomena, but the mechanisms that underlie this process have often been misinterpreted throughout humanity's eventful history. Perhaps the not-quite-cosmic-compensatory principle that things appear to even out over time could be termed 'the call of the mild'!

An example of 'the call of the mild' is the situation where the offspring of exceptionally intelligent, beautiful or talented parents tend to be slightly less intelligent, beautiful or talented than their parents. The good news for some of us is that the offspring of exceptionally unintelligent, plain and untalented parents also tend to be slightly less so than their parents. You might like to think of some real-life examples of this tendency for yourselves, or some exceptions to it (we are too aware of international libel

---

Box 10.2 **Regression towards exam mediocrity**

Quantitatively oriented lecturers often warn their students about to embark on examinations to be careful of 'regression towards the mean'. This does not necessarily indicate that the lecturers are worried about students becoming angry (mean) because they have stayed up all night studying, but that they should be wary of scores due partly to good or bad luck causing either false hopes or false disappointment.

To use a more positive example of regression towards the mean, you might have the bad luck to sit near someone who grunts and snorts throughout the exam, and so your marks will be lower than they should be, because examinations have a random component as well as measuring actual ability. In your next exam, it is (hopefully!) unlikely that you will sit next to the same grunting/snorting person, and so your mark might be a better reflection of your true ability, and so improve.[25]

An example of a suspected regression towards the mean in terms of measuring cognitive ability over time in Australian adolescents can be found in a recent study.[14] Further information on regression towards the mean, and on Sir Francis Galton himself, can be found in some recent articles in *Significance*.[26,27] This highly readable and enjoyable magazine (suitable for reading on a tram, train or bus) is a joint venture of the Royal Statistical Society and the American Statistical Association (see <www.significancemagazine.org>).

When designing or analysing the results of studies in which data are collected over time (and when sitting exams) please be careful of regression towards the mean (and good luck with your exams!).

laws to do this for you!). Galton himself considered that the process of intergenerational regression to the mean is attributable to the balancing genetic effects of grandparents and even earlier generations, but it is now considered likely that there is a random component to this process, as well as one that can be explained by genetics.

Conclusion

You have now completed 'Measures of association', parts one and two. An important message that you may like to take home, or somewhere else, after reading these two chapters on measures of association is that correlations tell us what goes with what, and regressions tell us what predicts or estimates what. The distinction between these tests of association is, however, really one of style rather than substance, as in practice you may well use either or both measures of association when possible — for example, when there are just two variables, such as height and weight.

Quick reference summary

- Regression differs from correlation in that it gives us a formula known as a regression equation that allows us to describe a predictive relationship between variables.

- This 'prediction' can be of concurrent variables such as depression and physical health levels, measured at the same point in time.

- As with most things, there are different types of regression. Some major types include simple linear regression, multiple regression, stepwise multiple regression, logistic regression and stepwise logistic regression.

- Which type of regression we should use will logically be determined by what we intend to use it for — the nature of the questions that we want to answer and the nature of our variables.

- Regression towards the mean has been interpreted by people of limited statistical literacy as a demonstration of a cosmic compensatory force, but it is actually more to do with the simple facts that things such as measures of human ability include a chance or random component, and that extremes are less likely to be followed by other extremes.

- Perhaps the not-quite-cosmic-compensatory principle that things appear to even out over time could be termed 'the call of the mild'.

References

1. Stigler SM. *The History of Statistics: the Measurement of Uncertainty before 1900*. Cambridge, MA: Harvard University Press; 1986.

2. Cohen J. Multiple regression as a general data-analytic system. *Psychological Bulletin*. 1968;70:426-443.

3. Cohen J, Cohen P, West SG, et al. *Applied Multiple Regression/ Correlation Analysis for the Behavioral Sciences*. 3rd ed. Mahwah, NJ: Erlbaum; 2003.

4. Tabachnick BG, Fidell LS. *Using Multivariate Statistics*. 6th ed. Upper Saddle River, NJ: Pearson; 2013.

5. Wright DB, London K. *Modern Regression Techniques Using R: a Practical Guide for Students and Researchers*. Thousand Oaks, CA: Sage; 2009.

6. Tu Y-K, Woolston A, Baxter PD, et al. Assessing the impact of body size in childhood and adolescence on blood pressure: an application of partial least squares. *Epidemiology*. 2010;21:440-448.

7. Efroymson MA. Multiple regression analysis. In: Ralston A, Wilf HS, eds. *Mathematical Methods for Digital Computers*. New York: Wiley; 1960:191-203.

8. Streiner DL. Regression in the service of the superego : the do's and don'ts of stepwise multiple regression. *Canadian Journal of Psychiatry*. 1994;39:191-196.

9. Derksen S, Keselman HJ. Backward, forward and stepwise automated subset selection algorithms: frequency of obtaining authentic and noise variables. *British Journal of Mathematical and Statistical Psychology*. 1992;45:265-282.

10. Kemp AH, Hopkinson PJ, Stephan BC, et al. Predicting severity of non-clinical depression: preliminary findings using an integrated approach. *Journal of Integrative Neuroscience*. 2006;5:89-110.

11. Billah B, Reid CM, Shardey GC, et al. A preoperative risk prediction model for 30-day mortality following cardiac surgery in an Australian cohort. *European Journal of Cardiothoracic Surgery*. 2010;37:1086-1092.

12. Mannan HR, McNeil JJ. Computer program to estimate overoptimism in measures of discordance for predicting the risk of cardiovascular disease. *Journal of Evaluation in Clinical Practice*. 2012, in press.

13. Austin PC. Bootstrap model selection had similar performance for selecting authentic and noise variables compared to backward variable elimination: a simulation study. *Journal of Clinical Epidemiology*. 2008;61:1009-1017.

14. Thomas S, Benke G, Dimitriadis C, et al. Use of mobile phones and changes in cognitive functioning in adolescents. *Occupational and Environmental Medicine*. 2010; 67:861-866.

15. Tait RS, French DJ, Hulse GK. Validity and psychometric properties of the General Health Questionnaire-12 in young Australian adolescents. *Australian and New Zealand Journal of Psychiatry*. 2003;37:374-381.

16. Savilla K, Kettler L, Galletly C. Relationships between cognitive deficits, symptoms and quality of life in schizophrenia. *Australian and New Zealand Journal of Psychiatry*. 2008;42:496-504.

17. Hosmer DW, Lemeshow S. *Applied Logistic Regression*. 2nd ed. New York: Wiley; 2000.

18. Clarke DM, Mackinnon AJ, Smith GC, et al. Dimensions of psychopathology in the medically ill: a latent trait approach. *Psychosomatics*. 2000;41:418-425.

19. McKenzie DP, Clarke DM, Forbes AB, et al. Pessimism, worthlessness, anhedonia, and thoughts of death identify DSM-IV major depression in hospitalized, medically ill patients. *Psychosomatics*. 2010;51:302-311.

20. Kelsall HL, McKenzie D, Sim MR, et al. Physical, psychological and functional comorbidities of multisymptom illness in Australian male veterans of the 1991 Gulf War. *American Journal of Epidemiology*. 2009;170:1048-1056.

21. Davies C, Corry K, Van Itallie A, et al. Prospective associations between interaction components and website engagement in a publicly available physical activity website: the case of 10,000 Steps Australia. *Journal of Medical Internet Research*. 2012;14:e4.

22. McKenzie M, Olsson CA, Jorm AF, et al. Association of adolescent symptoms of depression and anxiety with daily smoking and nicotine dependence in young adulthood: findings from a 10-year longitudinal study. *Addiction*. 2010;105:1642-1659.

23. Haller DM, Sanci LA, Patton GC, et al. Text message communication in primary care research: a randomized controlled trial. *Family Practice*. 2009;26:325-330.

24. Leverett FP. *Latin Lexicon: Latin–English and English–Latin*. Philadelphia, PA: Peter Reilly; 1931.

25. Shadish WR, Cook TD, Campbell DT. *Experimental and Quasi-experimental Designs for Generalized Causal Inference.* 2nd ed. Boston, MA: Houghton Mifflin; 2001.

26. Maier D. Francis Galton: measuring the immeasureable. *Significance.* 2011;8:122-123.

27. Senn S. Francis Galton and regression to the mean. *Significance.* 2011;8:124-126.

Further reading

Montgomery DC, Peck EA, Vining GG. *Introduction to Linear Regression Analysis.* 5th ed. New York: Wiley; 2012.

Norman GR, Streiner DL. *Biostatistics: the Bare Essentials.* 3rd ed. Hamilton, Ontario: BC Decker; 2008.

Steyerberg EW. *Clinical Prediction Models: a Practical Approach to Development, Validation and Updating.* New York: Springer; 2009.

CHAPTER 11

QUALITATIVE RESEARCH METHODS

The universe is made of stories, not atoms.
MURIEL RUKEYSER (1913–80)

Not everything that counts can be counted, and not everything that can be counted counts.
ALBERT EINSTEIN (1879–1955)

OBJECTIVES

After reading this chapter carefully you will:

- understand the nature of qualitative research and its associated analyses

- know how qualitative research and analysis differ from quantitative research and analysis

- be aware of some important advantages and disadvantages of qualitative research

- know when it is appropriate to use qualitative research

- understand when quality can be better than quantity.

Introduction

Some researchers working in at least some health sciences have an ongoing perception that there is a natural divide between qualitative research and quantitative research. As a result, health-science researchers and other health-science professionals tend to choose either qualitative or quantitative research (and subsequent analyses), in much the same way that we choose a political party to vote for, a football team to barrack for or a university to study or work in. In essence, however, the perceived distinction between these methods is often unnecessary and unhelpful. We do not need to choose one of them, with the implication that we have chosen it and no other, and that we are therefore either a qualitative or a quantitative researcher.

The choice of qualitative or quantitative research and statistical analysis should be made on the same basis as for the choice of any research method: it should be determined by the nature of the research question, rather than by rigid preconceptions or preferences. Whether or not you consider yourself to be a qualitative researcher, it is useful to have an open mind. Doing some qualitative research yourself at some stage or understanding the results of someone else's qualitative research may help to expand your current knowledge. It is actually possible and often useful to combine qualitative and quantitative research. The development of qualitative research is described in Box 11.1.

When to use qualitative research

There are situations in which qualitative research can offer health-science researchers important potential advantages over quantitative research. Qualitative research can be undertaken when we have small numbers of research participants. It also gives us great flexibility in the nature of the information we can obtain, and its interactive nature allow us to obtain 'deep' information. In many health-science research situations, information quality is more useful than information quantity; we are more interested in the different types of phenomena than in their number.

Qualitative research methodology can be appropriately and naturally employed when we do not have enough research cases to compare one experimental condition with others. In such situations useful research findings can still be obtained by analysing a few cases deeply instead of analysing many cases more summarily in an experimental design. A general example of this approach would be interviewing a small group of people to discover what issues related to our research interest are important to them. A specific example from the author's own health-science qualitative research experience involved the evaluation of an alcohol and other drug (AOD) harm minimisation program for young people.[1] Some of the information required for this evaluation was not suitable for an

---

Box 11.1 **Origins of qualitative research**

As with most statistical methods, qualitative analyses were not dreamed up in a contextual vacuum, but were developed to meet the needs of real research situations, just as the t-test was devised to help brewers brew better beer (see Chapter 7) and the ANOVA was devised to help farmers increase their wheat yields (see Chapter 8). Qualitative research was devised to meet the research needs of early anthropological and sociological researchers such as Bronislaw Malinowski (1884–1942) and Margaret Mead (1901–78), whose subject matter was not suited to quantitative analyses because of its inherent complexity and variability.

Early qualitative research was journalistic in style, in that it involved the unsystematic factual reporting of information. This information was typically presented by researchers in the form of reports of their observations and interviews in social settings where the action that interested them took place, such as in remote mountain villages or on city street corners.

More recently, qualitative research has become increasingly more systematic in its approach and has been influenced by theoretical approaches such as the symbolic interactionist perspective (which involves the belief that our social interactions give subjective meaning to human behaviour) and by grounded theory (which involves the ongoing generation of theory from data).

---

experimental approach or a quantitative analysis, because it came from a small number of key informants and it needed to be obtained interactively. Further relevant information was therefore acquired in interviews.

Qualitative research methodology can also be appropriately and naturally employed when there are many research cases, but we are interested in obtaining a deeper level of response information than would be possible with a purely quantitative approach. It is possible to conduct statistical analyses with large amounts of non-experimentally derived data using qualitative methods.

Mixed research designs

In situations where we need to understand or conduct research involving both qualitative and quantitative information, a research method using mixed (qualitative and quantitative) designs is used. These designs are becoming increasingly popular in health-science research because they can combine the objectivity of quantitative research with the flexibility and depth of analysis of qualitative research. The evaluation of the AOD harm reduction program mentioned above is an example of mixed-model research. A qualitative interview component was combined with a quantitative analysis of the aspects of the program that were better suited to it than to qualitative analysis, such as a comparison of the number of yearly episodes of care with that of yearly episodes of care targets.

Qualitative research in the health sciences

In the education and health-science fields, qualitative research methodology is increasingly applied more widely and systematically to answer research questions. Qualitative methods that were once mainly employed by anthropologists and sociologists have been adapted for use in these areas. Nursing, in particular, commonly uses qualitative research methods, but researchers in other health sciences such as psychology and medicine are also employing qualitative research more frequently.

As early as 1996, in a report by the British Psychological Society, there was a call for more qualitative psychological research to be undertaken.[2] In 1994, the first widely available qualitative research textbook was published in the UK[3] and the World Health Organization published an overview of the concepts and methods used in qualitative analysis.[4] A more recent description of the health-science related advantages of qualitative research appeared in 2000.[5]

Qualitative research can be a research rose of any other name, including 'case-study research', but, whatever its name, it is increasingly used and accepted in research in a wide range of health sciences.

An example of qualitative research in medicine

Qualitative research methods can be particularly useful in medical research and therefore ultimately in medical practice. This form of research can answer medical questions that quantitative research has difficulty answering, such as why some people do not adhere to a treatment regimen even though it is potentially of great benefit to them, and why some healthcare interventions are successful, even if such successes are medically counterintuitive.

A good example of the qualitative approach to information collection in medical action is provided by a study undertaken at the Durham Veterans Affairs Medical Center in North Carolina.[6] This was a qualitative study of 209 patients, each of whom had a serious and life-threatening illness. The patients were asked 'What is your understanding of your illness?' in order to gather potentially clinically useful information about the patients' perceptions of their illness severity, information that was largely absent from the existing medical literature. Themes that were identified in the responses to the study's open question varied by diagnosis, with the responses of cancer patients more often including diagnostic details and prognosis, and those of non-cancer patients more often including symptoms and causality. The researchers concluded that the results of the qualitative research could be used as a foundation for the development of patient-centred communication strategies and of a mutual clinician–patient understanding of illness and its consequences.

An example of qualitative research in nursing

Qualitative research methods are becoming increasingly important in developing knowledge for evidence-based nursing practice. It allows a wide variety of questions to be answered relating to the nursing profession's concern with real human responses, to real health problems. An example of this approach comes from nursing research at the University of Technology in Sydney.[7] This qualitative research involved the extraction of themes relating to why nurses are attracted to and remain in aged care and dementia care, based on a qualitative thematic analysis of themes emerging in 226 relevant research articles. The conclusion was that the intrinsic rewards of the caring role are what is important to these nurses.

An example of qualitative research in psychology

A well-known example of the valuable use of qualitative research methods in psychology is the development of theories of a child's intellectual and moral development by the Swiss psychologist and philosopher Jean Piaget (1896–1980). Piaget thought that psychometric testing was not capable of describing a child's innermost beliefs and reasoning processes, so he developed a qualitative methodology based on interviewing children. Piaget's approach concentrated on a richness of observation of a few cases (including his own children), rather than on a quantitative analysis of many cases.

One of Piaget's best-known theories is his conception of four discrete stages of intellectual development, culminating in the ability to think hypothetically. An accomplishment of early development famously described by Piaget is known as 'object permanence', in which infants of about 18 months of age are predicted to develop the understanding that although an object is covered it is still there. About a year ago, the author attempted his own informal empirical appraisal of this theory of cognitive development by placing a blanket over a ball in view of his then approximately 9-month-old daughter. Despite Piaget's theory that object permanence does not occur until about 18 months of age, Miranda knew what the blanket was covering, and removed it to get the ball underneath (Fig 11.1). Although there has been some scientific (and unscientific!) disagreement with at least some aspects of Piaget's theories, they still inform educational practices internationally.

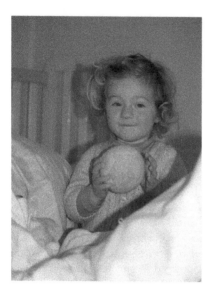

Fig 11.1 **Children aged over 18 months can easily find a ball under a blanket, as Miranda shows in this re-enactment of her demonstration of Piaget's object permanence theory when she was much younger.**

Common characteristics of qualitative methods

Some common characteristics of qualitative research are that it:

- tends to involve everyday situations rather than experimentally constructed ones

- involves a close relationship between the researcher and those being researched, such as via an interview or questionnaire

- is driven by those being researched rather than by the researcher, in that it can be open-ended and is guided by perceptions and interpretations other than those of the researcher

- is data-driven rather than theory-driven — research-related theory typically originates directly in the data rather than leading to its generation

- involves a detailed subjective description, qualitative analysis and interpretation of data

- is interactive — data collection and qualitative analysis typically proceed together and inform each other.

Qualitative research methods

The interview

The most commonly used qualitative research methodology is the interview. This typically consists of an interactive situation where the information provided by the interview respondent can shape the nature of further information that is obtained, such as when they indicate their particular interest. It is possible that an interviewee will provide information that the researcher did not expect, and a good interviewer can follow up on such potential leads by asking appropriate supplementary questions that will result in further relevant information being offered.

Good interviews often include initial questions that allow interviewees to provide information that is relevant to the researcher's particular interest, and also give interviewees opportunities to add to this information. The qualitative research interview could be described as a 'conversation with a purpose' and typically is used to elicit subjective information from the interviewee. Qualitative research interviews can be either formal or informal, and structured or unstructured. Interviews can be used as the main source of data collection or in conjunction with other forms of data gathering, including quantitative forms.

Formal and informal interviews

The 'in-depth interview' is intended to provide the interviewee with an opportunity to provide 'rich' subjective data, which means data that give an in-depth insight into those of the respondent's perspectives, perceptions, feelings and beliefs that are relevant to the researcher's interest. This type of interview is also known as the 'intensive interview'. Interviews can be formal or informal, but there is generally not a clear-cut distinction between these types. Formal interviews can be conducted with an individual or a group of individuals, and are more likely than informal interviews to be planned in advance and to be recorded. Informal interviews are more conversational and can take place when a researcher would like to further explore issues that have become apparent during some form of interaction with a potential interviewee, such as observing them.

Structured and unstructured interviews

Interviews can be unstructured, semi-structured or structured. An *unstructured interview* typically begins with a broad open question that generally relates to the area of research interest, such as: 'What do you think about … ?', or 'How do you feel about … ?'. This type of interview is typically driven by the interviewee, whose responses will determine the nature of subsequent questions. Interviewers also need to play an active part in the interview process, and typically do this by reminding interviewees (and themselves!) of the relevant research area, in order to keep the interview focused on it. Interviewers also typically use prompts, such as those often employed by journalists, psychotherapists, friends and other regular conductors of unofficial informal interviews — for example, 'Would you like to tell me more about that?' and 'How do you feel about that?'

Unstructured interviews are usually best suited to situations where little is known about the area of research interest, and can be used as the basis for the development of more structured methods of obtaining qualitative and quantitative information. The unstructured interview can be seen as the research equivalent of an 'ad lib' performance, where it is necessary for the performer to be continuously intuitively and spontaneously relevant to the topic.

Semi-structured and structured interviews rely more on scripted questions than on intuition and are therefore more closely related to a specific research agenda. Although these types of interviews are more focused on a research area than are unstructured interviews — and are sometimes known as 'focused interviews' — it is still important for the interviewer to be able to ask appropriate follow-up questions when necessary. As with the unstructured interview, in the semi-structured and structured interview the interviewee drives the interview process by answering questions in their own time and in their own words, but their responses are being elicited by specific questions. Structured and semi-structured interviews differ in their degree of adherence to a list of questions (a script), but in all types of qualitative interview there will be an opportunity for respondents to describe feelings and thoughts in their own words.

The questionnaire

Questionnaires are related to interviews in that they are designed and administered in order to elicit appropriate answers to appropriate research questions. Perhaps unsurprisingly, therefore, a questionnaire generally consists of a list of questions. Unlike the questions that are presented in an interview, which are typically presented verbally by the interviewer and answered verbally by the interviewee, a questionnaire is more commonly presented and answered in written form.

The advantage that questionnaires have over interviews is that they are relatively quick and easy to administer and can easily be given to large numbers of respondents simultaneously, including via the mail or internet, as well as in person. Interviews on the other hand can elicit a deeper level of response than questionnaires and give their respondents the opportunity of providing information that may not have been considered by the researcher. The comparative advantages and disadvantages of questionnaires and interviews are in a sense analogous to those of quantitative and qualitative research in general; indeed, questionnaires can be either fully quantitative, fully qualitative or a combination of the two, depending on the nature of their questions.

Questionnaire items can be designed to elicit a yes/no response, or a choice of responses that can indicate degrees of agreement, such as those measured by a Likert Scale (often containing five or seven response choices). A response of '1' might indicate information such as 'This statement doesn't apply to me at all', and a response of '7' might indicate information such as 'This statement applies strongly to me'. Questionnaire items can also elicit qualitative information, such as when they include spaces for respondents to record their beliefs and/or feelings on an issue in their own words.

It is possible to combine quantitative and qualitative analysis in a questionnaire by including both quantitative and qualitative items. Such combined or mixed designs can gather information that combines the objectivity and ease of analysis of quantitative information with the flexibility and depth of qualitative information. It is also possible to further relate quantitative and qualitative research in a questionnaire by asking respondents to provide contact details if they would like to provide further information in a subsequent interview.

Other qualitative research methods

Focus groups are a variant of research interviews. A group of people who may be able to provide input relevant to a research question are invited to come together and provide information in a structured or unstructured format, with varying degrees of adherence to a set of guiding questions. This is basically a 'think tank' that conceptually resembles quantitative test item development — a process that typically begins with the suggestion by people with relevant knowledge of possible test items, which will subsequently be tested and refined.

Unobtrusive methods are also commonly used in qualitative research and these generally consist of situations that do not require the active participation of those who are being researched. Examples of this form of qualitative research include going through existing sources, such as written records, or observations of human behaviour. These procedures are conceptually related to obtaining information from a clinical case history, which may include information that has not been directly obtained from the clinical case.

Thematic analysis

Identifying themes is central to qualitative research, but the understanding of just what constitutes a theme can vary. A theme is a construct and therefore a theoretical entity, and as such its usefulness depends on its ability to explain and to predict relevant phenomena. Basically, a theme is a story being told by the data and emerges in the form of commonalities of responses across many respondents. Examples of themes are seen in the previously mentioned qualitative medical study,[6] in which patients with serious illnesses were asked, 'What is your understanding of your illness?' Five major response themes were identified by the study authors: naming the diagnosis, the illness history, the prognosis, the symptoms and the causality.

Interview and questionnaire qualitative data can be analysed by the application of a thematic analysis, which can be either formal or informal. Thematic analysis basically consists of identifying common themes related to the research questions in the responses to interview or questionnaire questions. Formal thematic analysis is undertaken by running thematic analysis computer programs, while in informal thematic analysis the qualitative analyst goes through the data, identifies common responses and then determines the themes that they represent. To assist interpretation, findings are typically presented in tables that list the themes and the frequency of each thematic response.

Conceptually, the qualitative thematic analysis process can be seen as resembling the quantitative cluster analysis process, in which data that are considered to be similar on the basis of various objective criteria are computationally clustered (joined) to make larger units of data. An example of a thematic analysis is included in the combined qualitative/quantitative research example given below.

Qualitative statistical packages

Computer packages have been specifically developed to allow qualitative analysis, notably NVivo,[8] which along with its predecessor NUD*IST was developed in Melbourne.

Example of combined health-science research

Background

The author once designed a series of questionnaires that were intended to elicit qualitative and quantitative information about medical students' and psychology students' knowledge of, and attitudes towards, mindfulness as a clinical intervention for a range of conditions including anxiety and depression.[9,10] These questionnaires were administered to (a) medical students who had been exposed to a mindfulness education component in their course, (b) medical students without exposure to a mindfulness education component and (c) psychology students without exposure to a mindfulness education component.

The questionnaire consisted of 12 quantitative and qualitative items, including combined quantitative and qualitative items, which gave a total of 9 quantitative measures and 10 qualitative measures. Three of the 9 quantitative items used a five-point Likert scale that included item choices such as knowledge of mindfulness: (1) 'non-existent', (2) 'mild',

(3) 'moderate', (4) 'good' and (5) 'extensive'. Five of the 9 quantitative items utilised yes or no choice questions, such as 'Are there any clinical conditions that mindfulness might be useful for treating?' Four of the qualitative items were open-ended and invited the questionnaire respondents to comment on what makes mindfulness treatment suitable or unsuitable for the particular clinical conditions — anxiety, depression and substance abuse — and to comment on how mindfulness compares with other therapies such as cognitive behavioural therapies.

Results

The quantitative data obtained in this study were analysed using chi-square, logistic regression and Spearman's correlations. The results of the quantitative analysis showed that, perhaps as expected, medical students who were exposed to a mindfulness education component had a greater knowledge of mindfulness and a more positive attitude towards it (as measured by an increased willingness to administer or recommend it) than did medical students without a mindfulness component in their course, or psychology students without exposure to mindfulness in their course. The quantitative results also showed that these differences were substantial, as well as statistically significant, and that across students there was a significant and also strong relationship between knowledge of mindfulness and willingness to administer or refer it as treatment.

The qualitative data obtained in this study were analysed using an informal thematic method, whereby commonly emerging themes in the questionnaire responses were described for each of the student groups to demonstrate consistencies in responses. The results of this analysis added an explanatory dimension to the quantitative research findings that the three groups differed statistically, by describing *how* the three student groups differed in their knowledge of and attitude towards mindfulness, and to what extent.

The most common response themes that emerged in the qualitative analysis for the psychology students without exposure was that mindfulness is useful as a treatment because: (1) it reduces people's stress; (2) it is a non-medical treatment that does not produce side effects; (3) it is suitable for a wide range of people; and (4) it improves people's mental state. The most common and only response theme that emerged for the medical students without exposure to mindfulness was that they do not know enough about it to have an opinion on its usefulness. The most common response themes that emerged for the medical students exposed to mindfulness was that it is useful as a clinical treatment because: (1) it helps improve people's overall health and wellbeing; (2) it reduces people's stress; (3) it is inexpensive; and (4) there is research that supports its usefulness. This research example demonstrates how qualitative and quantitative research and analysis can be combined in a complementary and productive research relationship.

Pros and cons of qualitative and quantitative research

Qualitative research

A major advantage of qualitative research methods is that they allow research participants to provide the researcher with rich and interactive information. The closer relationship between researcher and researched in the qualitative research context makes it possible for the research participant to offer in-depth information, which can result in a more genuine and deeper level of communication with research participants than is possible in quantitative research.

When research participants are being asked for their own answer, in their own words, they can potentially reveal a level of information that may not be possible with numeric scores or forced-choice selections. Information obtained by qualitative methodologies could be likened to tailor-made clothes, where the research respondent is listened to attentively and the information-gathering process is individually suited to their responses. Information obtained by quantitative methodologies could be likened to off-the-peg clothes, or even to one-size-fits-all clothes. Many quantitative researchers have been faced with the uncomfortably naked truth of situations where their research participants have stated forlornly that 'none of the choices you offered me was the answer that I wanted to give!'

A major disadvantage of qualitative research methods is that they can be subjective, which makes it difficult to compare results between people, locations and researchers. Qualitative testing can also be complex and therefore more expensive and time-consuming to administer than quantitative methodologies.

Quantitative research

Major advantages of quantitative research methods are that they are objective and relatively quick to administer and interpret, with research results expressed only in numbers that are easy to standardise so that researchers across research sites and research areas can meaningfully compare their scores.

A major disadvantage of using quantitative research methods is that they can result in information and rich detail being missed. In Chapter 2, 'Statistics as Information', we pointed out that when information measurement scales are used to reduce information, or when information is deliberately reduced to fewer information units, we lose information. This is generally true of quantitative as opposed to qualitative information, in that qualitative information is inherently more detailed. Obtaining or preserving such information richness, however, can result in problems such as a lack of standardisation and objectivity.

A health-science example

In the 1950s, two main approaches to neuropsychological testing emerged approximately concurrently, each with advantages and disadvantages that are conceptually similar to those of qualitative and quantitative research methodologies. Psychometric (numbers-based) neuropsychological testing was developed primarily in North America, where it is still widely used. A more intuitive approach appeared in Europe, and is still widely used there, which originated in the work of theorists such as Rey in France and Luria in what was then the USSR. These theorists could be seen as being more concerned with the 'why', or underlying nature, of neuropsychological conditions than with the 'what' of their associated quantitative scores. In Australia a combination of the psychometric and the more intuitive approaches tends to be used. This combined approach could be considered the equivalent of the mixed-model qualitative/quantitative research approach — a balanced approach that combines the advantages of both of its components.

Conclusion

Doing qualitative or quantitative research is not an either/or choice — you do not have to sign up for one camp or the other, or take life-long vows of loyalty. If you choose to do qualitative research, it will not necessarily make you a lifelong qualitative researcher, and therefore as unwelcome at quantitative research functions as a Guelph would have been at a Ghibelline function in renaissance Italy, or vice versa. (Incidentally, this historical example of opposing camps is probably what inspired Shakespeare to write about the romantic/political/family problems that were experienced by Romeo and Juliet, and even more incidentally by Maria and Tony in the twentieth-century New York version, *West Side Story*.)

As you might have realised by now, it is possible, even praiseworthy, to simultaneously conduct qualitative and quantitative research, because, as in any great and lasting relationship, the two components can together attain something greater than the sum of the individual parts. Qualitative research is completely different from but not incompatible with quantitative research, it can provide important insights into health-related phenomena and it can inform and enrich further research.

Quick reference summary

- You do not have to choose between doing qualitative or quantitative research; you can (legally and valuably) do both.

- The choice between doing qualitative or quantitative research should be driven by your research question, not your self-image.

- Qualitative research can help us find out the different types of things that exist rather than the amount of them.

- Qualitative research can be undertaken when we have small numbers of research participants; it can give us great flexibility in the nature of the information obtained using it, and we can obtain 'deep' information as a result of its interactive nature.

- Qualitative research methods include the interview, the questionnaire and thematic analysis.

- Qualitative research can provide important insights into health-related phenomena, and can inform and enrich further research.

References

1. McKenzie S, Droste N, Miller P. Reducing alcohol and other drug related harm in young people: evaluation of a youth engagement program. *Youth Studies Australia*. 2011;30(4):51-59.

2. Richardson J, ed. *Handbook of Qualitative research Methods for Psychology and the Social Sciences*. Leicester: British Psychological Society; 1996.

3. Bannister P, Bruman E, Parker I, et al. *Qualitative Methods in Psychology: a Research Guide*. Milton Keynes: Open University Press; 1994.

4. Hudelson P. *Qualitative Research for Health Programs, Division of Mental Health*. Geneva: World Health Organization; 1994.

5. Winch PJ, Wagman JA, Maloouin RA, et al. *Qualitative Research for Improved Health Programs. A Guide to Manuals for Qualitative and Participatory Research on Child Health, Nutrition, and Reproductive Health*. Baltimore: Department of International Health, Johns Hopkins University, School of Hygiene and Public Health; 2000. Available online at <http://sara.aed.org/publications/cross_cutting/qualitative/qualitative.pdf>. Accessed 1 October 2012.

6. Morris DA, Johnson KS, Ammarell N, et al. What is your understanding of your illness? A communication tool to explore patients' perspectives of living with advanced illness. *Journal of General Internal Medicine*. 2012. [Epub 26 May ahead of print]

7. Chenoweth L, Jeon Y, Merlyn T, et al. A systematic review of what factors attract and retain nurses in aged and dementia care. *Journal of Clinical Nursing*. 2010;19(1–2):156-167.

8. NVivo website: <http://www.qsrinternational.com/products_nvivo.aspx>.

9. McKenzie S, Hassed C, Gear L. Medical and psychology students' knowledge of and attitudes towards mindfulness as a clinical intervention: a comparison of students with and without exposure to mindfulness in their course. *Explore*. 2012;8(6):360-367.

10. McKenzie S, Hassed C. *Mindfulness for Life*. Wollombi: Exisle; 2012.

CHAPTER 12

STATISTICS IN
THE HEALTH SCIENCES

*[Statistics are] the only tools by which an opening can be cut
through the formidable thicket of difficulties that bar the path
of those who pursue the Science of Man.*

SIR FRANCIS GALTON (1822–1911)

OBJECTIVES

After carefully reading this chapter you will understand:

- the special statistical needs of the health sciences

- the nature and application of some statistics that are
  especially relevant to the health sciences

- how some health-science statistics differ from, or are
  similar to, other commonly used statistics.

Introduction

As you may have realised by now, statistics are vital to health-science research and practice in a wide range of health sciences, including medicine, nursing, psychology, pharmacy, radiography and health policy. The statistical methods we have discussed up to this point are general methods that are commonly used in the health sciences as well as in many other situations. This chapter will introduce you to statistics that could be considered specific to the health sciences, in that they are used more often in the health sciences than in other areas. Many of the general principles you have learned in the context of general statistics also apply to these health-science statistics, such as the importance of looking at effect sizes and confidence intervals rather than just at statistical significance.

Research is commonly undertaken and interpreted in the health sciences. It plays an important role in the development of clinical treatments and tests, and in the identification of areas of health need. Research supports clinical practice and administration by generating vital information about the safety and efficacy of drugs and other treatments, and checking the accuracy of clinical tests, whether they are new physiological and psychometric tests in development or well-established ones.

This chapter will introduce you to some practical statistical principles and techniques specific to the health sciences, including some that have particular clinical relevance, in that they directly concern condition diagnosis and prognosis. These principles and techniques will be illustrated by health-science examples, including clinical ones. This chapter will also present descriptions of test sensitivity and specificity, positive and negative predictive power, and odds ratios and relative risk.

Effect size and sample characteristics

The importance of looking at effect size, confidence intervals and statistical significance when performing and interpreting statistical analyses has already been mentioned in several contexts. This is particularly important in health-science research, and especially clinical research. In clinical situations more than in many other situations, the statistical proof is contained in the statistical pudding. A statistically significant improvement between one treatment and another, or between treatment and no treatment, for example, may be meaningless if there is no corresponding clinical benefit.

In health-science research, as in the use and interpretation of general statistical methods, it is vital to consider sample size. Is the sample size so large that almost any statistical result — no matter how minuscule — will be statistically significant? Is the sample size so small that we cannot make meaningful inferences from it about the population that interests us? Health-science statistical applications and interpretation can be particularly hazardous for the statistically ignorant (statistical pagans) or misguided (statistical heathens). It is therefore important to chart and steer a middle path between potential rocks (Scylla) and hard places (Charybdis) — actually whirlpools. This means we should always look at the magnitude and practical importance of our results, and at the characteristics of the sample on which they were based.

It is also important that the sample is truly representative of the population that interests us. Did every member of that population have an equal chance of being in our sample? In addition, we need to be clear about the definition of the population that underlies our sample (determining this is not always as easy as introductory statistics books have sometimes suggested).

In the real health-science world, well-meaning statistical advice often enters one statistically semi-literate ear and soon leaves through the other one, without troubling the central executive processing capacity that is reputed to exist between them. If, however, we can constantly remember the reason for doing the right thing, statistically speaking, we will be more likely to do it than if we just robotically follow statistical laws, for a while.

Diagnostic statistics

What sorts of clinical decisions do you think that somebody working in the health sciences might need to make? Clinical decisions are not only made by the people who work in a clinical setting; many other people need to interpret clinical results for indirect clinical purposes, such as allocating clinical resources. It is common for people working clinically, either directly or indirectly, to have to make decisions — or to be involved in decision-making processes — about what level of functioning people may have, and whether or not they have a health-affecting impairment or condition. There are statistical techniques and principles that relate specifically to clinical diagnosis, and some of the particularly relevant and useful ones will be described here.

Types of diagnostic error

If we make a clinical diagnosis, there are two ways that we can be right, and there are two ways that we can be wrong. A clinical diagnosis therefore provides four possible information conditions, which can be shown in a two-by-two table (Table 12.1). This table could be seen as conceptually

TABLE 12.1 DIAGNOSTIC TEST POSSIBILITIES

	Diagnostic test result	
Actual disease/disorder	True positive	False negative
	False positive	True negative

related to the two-by-two table that we used to illustrate the application of a chi-square test in Chapter 7.

If we diagnose a woman with a condition (such as pregnancy) that she actually has (i.e. she *is* pregnant), then we are correct, and this diagnostic information can be described as a true positive. If we diagnose a woman as not having a condition (such as pregnancy) that she does not have (she *is not* pregnant), then we are also correct, and this can be described as a true negative. All is therefore well, so far. If we diagnose a woman as having a condition (such as pregnancy) that she does not have (she *is not* pregnant), then we have made a diagnostic error. This (dis)information can be described as a false positive (or 'crying wolf', in slightly less technical language). If we diagnose a woman as not having a condition (such as pregnancy) that she does have (she *is* pregnant), then we have made a diagnostic error. This (dis)information can be described as a false negative. In the latter two cases, all is therefore not quite so well.

In a perfect clinical world there are no diagnostic errors, but we are not currently living, working or performing statistical analyses in such a world, so diagnostic errors do exist. It is therefore clinically vital to pragmatically manage and reduce the potential harm of diagnostic errors. The first guiding principle of clinical statistics, and of statistics in general, may well be the same as the first guiding rule of medicine: 'First, do no harm'!

There are clinical situations where it is particularly important not to make false positive diagnostic errors, and there are others where it is particularly important not to make false negative diagnostic errors. Clinical statistics called sensitivity/specificity analyses (and the related positive and negative predictive power analyses) allow us to trade off between our false negative and false positive rates, according to clinical need. Positive and negative predictive values, as well as sensitivity and specificity values, can be generated based on the two ways that we can be right when we make a clinical diagnosis (true positives and true negatives) and the two ways that we can be wrong (false positives and false negatives). Positive and negative predictive values give us a different view of our pattern of diagnostic errors from the pattern that is given by sensitivity and specificity values.

We can use the sensitivity/specificity and positive/negative predictive power analyses, as well as hit rates, to calculate a test's diagnostic performance, and use this information to inform appropriate modifications of our testing interpretation procedure, such as by altering the level of our diagnostic criteria for stating whether a condition is present or absent.

Sensitivity

In which clinical testing situation do you think that it is particularly important to minimise false negatives (that is, telling people that they do not have a condition when in fact they do have it)? A low false-negative rate is vital when we are screening for a condition. For example, if we are screening the population of an entire school or a group of schools to identify possible cases of an infectious disease, we do not want to miss potential cases. In this situation we must set our diagnostic bar at a height that will allow the identification of all possible cases, which means lowering our false-negative rate. Other relevant examples of this process would be screening children for vision or hearing problems, and screening adults for breast and bowel cancer.

The false-negative/false-positive trade-off means that as we have fewer false negatives (people who have an infectious disease/hearing or vision problem/breast or bowel cancer whom we diagnose as not having the condition), we will also have more false positives (people who do not have a condition that we are screening for and whom we diagnose as having it). In screening situations such as this, decreasing our false-negative rate at the expense of increasing our false-positive rate is appropriate, because further testing of the possible cases identified may reveal whether the false positives are indeed false positives. The vital requirement in this testing situation is *not to miss possible cases*.

Sensitivity can be regarded as the detection rate of a test. The higher the sensitivity of a test, the lower its false negative rate will be, and therefore the higher its true positive rate. The sensitivity rate of a test can be calculated by dividing the number of true positives obtained by the number of true positives plus false negatives obtained — in other words, the number of people who have the condition and who test positive divided by the number of people who have the condition.

$$\text{Sensitivity} = \frac{\text{true positives}}{\text{true positives} + \text{false negatives}}$$

Specificity

In which clinical testing situation do you think that it is important to minimise false positives (that is, telling people they have a condition when in fact they do not)? When we are providing a conclusive diagnosis, especially if it relates to a condition that can involve serious treatment or life consequences, such as severe chronic depression[1] or pregnancy, it is important not to tell somebody that they have a condition when in fact they do not. In this situation it is better to set the diagnostic bar at a height that may not allow the diagnosis of all possible cases, which means lowering our false positive rate.

The false-negative/false-positive trade-off means that we will have fewer false positives (people who do not have severe chronic depression or who are not pregnant, but whom we diagnose as having the condition) but we will have more false negatives (people who do have the condition and whom we diagnose as not having it). Decreasing our false-positive rate at the expense of increasing our false-negative rate is appropriate in this case, because it is important not to precipitate invasive treatments or life changes for people who do not have the condition we are diagnosing.

Specificity can be seen as the misdiagnosis rate of a test or, in slightly less technical language, the number of times 'wolf' is cried. The higher the specificity of a test, the lower the false positive rate, and therefore the higher the true negative rate. The specificity of a test can be calculated by dividing the number of true negatives obtained by the number of true negatives plus false positives or, in other words, the number of people who do not have the condition and who test negative, divided by the number of people who do not have the condition.

$$\text{Specificity} = \frac{\text{true negatives}}{\text{true negatives} + \text{false positives}}$$

Positive predictive power

The positive predictive value of a test is the chance that a positive test result will be correct or, to express this in another way, the probability that the test will be correct when we predict that the condition that interests us is present.

A test's positive predictive value can be calculated by dividing the true positives obtained by true positives plus false positives. In other words the proportion of true positives is given by the number of people who test positive and who actually have the disease or disorder, divided by the number of people who test positive.

$$\text{Positive predictive value} = \frac{\text{true positives}}{\text{true positives} + \text{false positives}}$$

Negative predictive power

The negative predictive value of a test is the chance that a negative test result will be correct or, to express this in another way, the probability that a test will be correct if it predicts that the condition that interests us is absent.

A test's negative predictive value can be calculated by dividing true negatives obtained by true negatives plus false negatives. In other words, the proportion of true negatives is given by the number of people who test negative and who do not have the disease or disorder divided by number of people who test positive.

$$\text{Negative predictive value} = \frac{\text{true negatives}}{\text{true negatives} + \text{false negatives}}$$

Hit rates

The overall predictive power or diagnostic accuracy of a test is its *hit rate*. This can be calculated by adding the true positives obtained to the true negatives obtained, and dividing the result of this by the sum of its true positives, false negatives, false positives and true negatives (or true positives plus true negatives divided by total number of people).

$$\text{Hit rate} = \frac{\text{true positives} + \text{true negatives}}{\text{number of people tested}}$$

ROC curves

If you know something about ornithology or mythology (or both), you might think that a ROC is a large and often angry bird. It is actually a computational technique that can be used for calculating trade-offs between a test's sensitivity and its specificity at different test cut-off points, and ROC stands for Receiver Operating Characteristic. The ROC curve was developed at about the time of the Second World War by electrical engineers as a means of tracking enemy planes on radar and by experimental psychologists working in perception. The ROC curve allows the creation of an optimal trade-off between sensitivity and specificity, depending on the purpose of the test, such as by using different clinical decision cut-off points.[2]

The ROC curve plots sensitivity on its *y* (vertical) axis, and 1 minus specificity on its *x* (horizontal) axis. For example, a test's true-positive rate at various cut-off points can be plotted on the *y* axis, and its false-positive rate at different cut-off points (expressed as 1 minus specificity) on the *x* axis. The area under the ROC curve can then be calculated, and this will be equal to the probability that a randomly chosen person who actually has the diagnosed disease has a higher value of the measurement (for example, a positive test result) than a randomly chosen person without the disease. The higher the area under the ROC curve, the better the diagnostic result, while an area under the curve of 0.50 represents chance level performance.[3]

There are various relatively simple and not-quite-so-simple methods for calculating the area under a ROC curve, including a non-parametric method that is related to the Mann-Whitney-Wilcoxon test that you encountered in Chapter 7. It is enough to tell you here, however, that ROC exists and what it does, without potentially ROCking your boat by explaining *how* it does it.

A ROC curve in flight

An example of using a sensitivity/specificity trade-off is the administration and interpretation of the MMSE cognitive screen.[4] Health-science workers in a number of areas, including medicine, psychiatry, nursing and psychology, usually use a score of 27/30 on this test as the diagnostic criterion (the point at which we usually define scores above this point as signifying that the condition (dementia) is absent), and define scores below this as signifying that the condition (dementia) is present. This is the level that has been generally found to provide maximum sensitivity as a cognitive screen, without reducing specificity too much. If we change the mini-mental status examination (MMSE) cut-off point to 26 or 25, we will increase the test's sensitivity by reducing its false-negative rate, but we will also decrease the test's specificity, by reducing its true-negative rate. Incidentally, cut-off points are dependent on place and time and it may not be possible to generalise them well from one country or time to another country or time.[5] A study has demonstrated this lack of generalisability for the 12-item version of the general health questionnaire (GHQ), a widely used measure of physical and psychological distress.[6,7]

A sensitivity/specificity analysis in clinical research action

When the author worked at the National Ageing Research Institute (North West Hospital/University of Melbourne) one of his research missions was to devise a better dementia diagnostic screen than was then available. The screening test battery that we devised consisted of selections of quantitative electroencephalographic (QEEG) measures, cued recall and selective reminding specific memory measures,[8] and the widely used cognitive screens — the MMSE[4] and the abbreviated mental test score (AMTS).[9]

Sensitivity and specificity levels were calculated for the newly devised screens on the basis of results obtained from their administration to a large number of people who had been clinically diagnosed with various forms of dementia. The gold standard that we used to assess the sensitivity and the specificity of the newly devised screens was a clinical diagnosis based on a comprehensive test battery, including MRI scan and neuropsychological testing.

The diagnostic sensitivity and specificity of the newly devised dementia screens were compared with the results obtained using the MMSE and AMTS combined for diagnosing a range of dementias, including Alzheimer's disease.[10,11,12] The memory and QEEG measures that were diagnostically most useful were selected on the basis of logistic regressions. The results of this analysis showed that dementia sensitivity and specificity levels for the newly developed measures were approximately equivalent to those obtained with the combined administration of the AMTS and the MMSE. Even more interestingly, the combined sensitivity and specificity levels of the AMTS and MMSE improved when the diagnostically best specific memory test measures were added to them; they were further improved when the best QEEG measures were added; and improved even further when the best 'cognitive challenge' QEEG measures were added. The 'cognitive challenge' consisted of creating a 'brain stress test' by asking research participants to count backwards while their brain waves were recorded.

In this way a dementia screen was devised that did not significantly increase the time taken to administer currently widely used cognitive screens, but that improved their diagnostic accuracy. This newly devised test therefore provided a diagnostic option (for one hospital at least) that lay between the brevity and simplicity of widely used cognitive screens, and the greater diagnostic accuracy offered by a clinical diagnosis based on a comprehensive evaluation.

Relative risks and odds ratios

In Chapter 10 you learned that regression analysis allows the prediction of the unknown based on the known. A commonly used example of this process is the weather. If it has been sunny and warm for the last three days, our best guess about the weather that is likely on the fourth day is that it will also be sunny and warm. Relative risk and odds ratios are statistical techniques that are particularly important in the health sciences, and they relate to the principles that underlie regression.

Relative risks and odds ratios provide health professionals and health policy analysts with information relating to the chances that individuals or groups of individuals will develop health problems, given their known risk factors. These clinical statistics are very useful, because they can give us vital information on the odds or risk of y (where y is a disease or consequence of a disease), given our knowledge of a person's scores on a range of relevant associated factors (x variables). Odds ratios are typically used with cross-sectional, case-control and/or retrospective data. Relative risk is typically used for randomised control trials (RCT) or prospective designs.

Odds ratios and relative risks relate to the chi-square and sensitivity/specificity/positive/negative predictive power analyses that we have covered above, in that they can also be described using two-by-two tables. The underlying concepts of the odds ratios and relative risk statistical techniques are, perhaps unsurprisingly, odds and risks. The relationship between these concepts has caused some confusion about their differences and similarities, and when it is appropriate to use each; examples of the calculations for both are provided in the following section.

A relative risk/odds ratio analysis

When the author worked in a Victorian Transcultural Psychiatry Unit (St Vincent's Hospital/University of Melbourne), one of his research missions was to determine to what extent the likelihood of adults from an English-speaking background (ESB) being admitted as psychiatric inpatients differed from that of adults from a non-English speaking background (NESB) in a predominantly English-speaking city (Melbourne). A non-English speaking background was defined as one where English was not

TABLE 12.2 CHANCES OF BEING ADMITTED AS A PSYCHIATRIC INPATIENT
IN ONE YEAR

Adults 15–64 years of age	Number admitted as psychiatric inpatients	Number NOT admitted as psychiatric inpatients	Total
ESB	6549	2,229,336	2,235,885
NESB	362	622,917	623,279
Total	6911	2,852,253	2,859,164

a person's preferred language, and being included as an 'adult' was based
on being between 15 and 64 years of age. People of 65 years of age and
over were included in a separate analysis as 'seniors'. The results of the
main analysis showed that in the same year 1 in 341 ESB people (6549
out of 2,235,885, or 0.003%) were admitted as psychiatric inpatients, but
1 in 1722 NESB people (362 out of 623,279, or 0.0006%) were admitted
(Table 12.2).[13] These two statistics can be called risk estimates, because
they describe the risk that an ESB and a NESB person has of being admitted as a psychiatric inpatient in the course of a year.

Risk estimates

The risk estimate difference in the above example is, perhaps not unexpectedly, the difference between our obtained risk estimates, which in this case
is 0.003% – 0.0006% = 0.0024%. The risk difference is not an ideal way
of describing the comparative risks between groups, because often these
involve such small numbers that the difference between them may appear
trivial, even if it is not trivial to the people experiencing the risk.

It is more useful to create a risk ratio of the risks that we are interested
in comparing, which is known as relative risk. This is calculated by applying the following formula, which is given, perhaps ironically in this
example, in English:

> *The risk of one event occurring relative to the risk of another event
> occurring is the risk of one event occurring divided by the risk of the
> other event occurring.*

Applying this formula, the risk of being admitted as a psychiatric inpatient
if you are from an ESB relative to your risk of being admitted as a psychiatric inpatient if you are from an NESB is 0.003 ÷ 0.0006 = 5. This
means that if you are from an ESB you are 5 times as likely to be admitted
as a psychiatric inpatient in a year as you are if you are from an NESB.

Odds ratios

Odds ratios are related to, but different from, relative risks, the difference
being that to calculate odds ratios we need to divide occurrences of an

event by non-occurrences of the event, rather than by the event total (occurrences plus non-occurrences) as we would for relative risk. The odds of somebody from an ESB or an NESB being admitted as a psychiatric inpatient can be expressed in English, more or less, as follows:

The odds of one event occurring relative to the odds of another event occurring is the odds of one event occurring divided by the odds of the other event occurring.

Applying this formula to our example, the odds of being admitted as a psychiatric inpatient if you are from an ESB is 0.003 ÷ 0.0006 = 5, which is the same as the relative risk. The sameness of the result is due to rounding, but if we had given the result with more decimal places we would have detected a very slight difference created by dividing occurrences by non-occurrences rather than dividing by the total, as for relative risk.

The bigger risk picture

Relative risks and odds ratio calculations provide us with similar results but they relate to slightly different underlying concepts. It is perhaps natural for us to consider that our risk of being admitted as a psychiatric inpatient if we are from an ESB is 0.003 of all people from an ESB, as in the relative risk calculation. It is perhaps less natural for us to consider that the odds of us being admitted as a psychiatric inpatient if we are from an ESB are 0.003 of people who are not admitted, as in the odds ratio calculation.

In this example both the relative risk and the odds ratios reveal that an 'adult' from an ESB is 5 times more likely than an 'adult' from an NESB to be admitted as a psychiatric inpatient. Does this (genuine) result therefore mean that people from an NESB background are 5 times saner than those from an ESB background? Does this result actually mean that people from a NESB have a similar sanity level to people from an ESB, but are 5 times less likely to utilise psychiatric services, possibly for reasons that relate to cross-cultural differences in attitudes towards mental illness and its treatment? Research funding to investigate these competing possible explanations further is still eagerly awaited!

Conclusion

You have been introduced in this chapter to some statistical methods that are commonly and valuably used in the health sciences in particular. As with all statistics, these health-science statistics need to be chosen, applied and interpreted appropriately and carefully. In Chapter 13 you will be introduced to some statistics that are not only very useful in the health sciences, but also in many other areas.

Quick reference summary

- Research is commonly undertaken and interpreted in the health sciences, and this research has a vital role in the development of clinical treatments and tests and in the identification of areas of health need.

- Statistical tests that are particularly relevant for the health sciences include tests that are used to assist clinical diagnosis and prognosis.

- A test's sensitivity can be seen as its detection rate.

- A test's specificity can be seen as its misdiagnosis rate.

- The positive predictive value of a test is the chance that a positive test result will be correct.

- The negative predictive value of a test is the chance that a negative test result will be correct.

- Relative risk is the risk of one event occurring relative to the risk of another event occurring.

- Odds ratios are the odds of one event occurring relative to the odds of another event occurring.

References

1. Horwitz AV, Wakefield JC. *The Loss Of Sadness: How Psychiatry Transformed Normal Sorrow into Depressive Disorder*. New York: Oxford University Press; 2007.

2. Swets JA. *Signal Detection Theory and ROC Analysis in Psychology and Diagnostics: Collected Papers*. Mahwah, NJ: Erlbaum; 1995.

3. Kraemer HC. *Evaluating Medical Tests: Objective and Quantitative Guidelines*. Newbury Park, CA: Sage; 1992.

4. Folstein MF, Folstein SE, McHugh PR. Mini-mental state. A practical method for grading the cognitive state of patients for the clinician. *Journal of Psychiatric Research*. 1975;12(3): 189-198.

5. Donath S. The validity of the 12-item General Health Questionnaire in Australia: a comparison between three scoring methods. *Australian and New Zealand Journal of Psychiatry*. 2001;35:231-235.

6. Goldberg DP, Williams P. *A User's Guide to the General Health Questionnaire*. Windsor, Berks: NFER-Nelson; 1988.

7. Goldberg DP, Oldehinkel T, Ormel J. Why GHQ threshold varies from one place to another. *Psychological Medicine.* 1998;28:915-921.

8. Bushke H. Selective Reminding analysis of memory and learning. *Journal of Verbal Learning and Verbal Behaviour.* 1973;12:543-550.

9. Hodkinson HM. Evaluation of a mental test score for assessment of mental impairment in the elderly. *Age and Ageing.* 1972;1(4):233-238.

10. McKenzie S, Yates M, Jenkin R, et al. Multi-channel quantitative EEG (QEEG) in the diagnosis of incipient dementia. *Australian Geriatric Society Conference, Adelaide.* 1992.

11. McKenzie S, Flicker L, Jenkin R, et al. Multi-channel quantitative EEG (QEEG) in the diagnosis of Alzheimer's type dementia. *Australian Association of Gerontology Conference, Adelaide.* 1993.

12. McKenzie S, Flicker L, Ames D. Multi-channel quantitative EEG (QEEG) and memory testing in the diagnosis of dementia. *Australian Psychological Society, Special Interest Group on Ageing Conference, Melbourne.* 1996.

13. Klimidis S, Lewis J, Miletic T, et al. *Mental Health Service Use by Ethnic Community in Victoria.* Melbourne: Victorian Transcultural Psychiatry Unit/Centre for Cultural Studies and Research; 1999.

Further reading

Howell D C. *Statistical Methods for Psychology.* 7th ed. Belmont, CA: Wadsworth; 2010.

CHAPTER 13

RELIABILITY, VALIDITY AND NORMS

OBJECTIVES

After carefully reading this chapter you will know:

- what reliability is
- what validity is
- what norms are
- how being familiar with these concepts can help you to better understand health-science testing and test results.

Introduction

Clinical research undertaken and interpreted in the health sciences often relates to the results of clinical tests. Clinical tests that are commonly used include new physiological and psychometric tests that are being developed, as well as established tests such as blood pressure and IQ. In order to determine just how good a new or existing clinical test is, we need to know about some of its important characteristics, such as its reliability, validity and norms.

We can illustrate the difference between reliability and validity with an archery example. If we shoot a series of arrows at a target and they each hit it in the same spot, this is reliability; if they each hit the bulls-eye, this is validity. A physics example can be used to illustrate what norms are. According to Einstein's theory of relativity, things are only meaningful in relation to other things. Similarly, a norm is a characteristic of many test scores that becomes meaningful when compared with a particular test score. These preliminary definitions will be elaborated in the following sections.

Reliability

What makes a test of blood pressure or IQ or even statistics knowledge reliable? If you are thinking of an answer that is very complicated, or if you are not thinking of anything at all, then smilingly move on, as ever. The technical meaning of reliability is exactly the same as the everyday meaning of reliability and can be defined as constancy, or consistency (Fig 13.1).

A reliable clinical test is much the same as a reliable car or friend — we can generally trust it to be constant. A reliable test is one that provides us with consistent measures, either across time or at a single point in time. A test that is fully reliable over time is one that gives us the same results at a point in the future as it does today. A test that is fully reliable at a single point in time is one in which people score in the same way on different parts of a test.

Reliability relates to the characteristics of the probability sampling distribution described by the central limit theorem (introduced in Chapter 2 and mentioned again in Chapter 4). As a result of these characteristics, generally the more items that are contained in a test, the more reliable it will be.

The higher the reliability coefficient of a test, the more reliable it is. Reliability coefficients vary between 0 and 1. A reliability coefficient of 1 means that a test has perfect reliability — that is, there is total consistency between different administrations of the test, or between administrations of different parts of the test. A reliability coefficient of 0 means that a test has no reliability. A factor that can reduce the reliability of a test is testing error, so the more instances of testing error there are in a test (that is, the

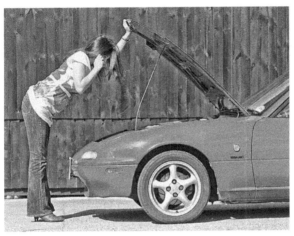

Fig 13.1   Unreliability — both statistical and general (Robert Grounds/Flickr)

more fluctuations in scores due to factors other than the actual character-istics of interest to the test taker), the less reliable it is.

A test's reliability can be measured by reliability-related applications of the correlation statistics that were introduced in Chapter 9, which can be used to provide reliability correlation coefficients. The reliability coeffi-cient was developed independently by Spearman[1] (of Spearman's correla-tion fame) and Brown[2] in 1910 for calculating the reliability of multivariate psychological tests. These coefficients later flourished and evolved into several related types of test reliabilities that are commonly calculated: inter-rater reliability, test–retest reliability and split-half reliability.

Inter-rater reliability

This is a measure of the reliability among different raters of test phenom-ena such as the tastiness of wines or cheeses or the efficacy of clinical treatments. A health-science example of a test that generally has a low inter-rater reliability is the Rorschach inkblot test. The basic idea behind the development and application of this test is that our inner conflicts can influence our interpretations of ambiguous stimuli, such as inkblots. A 2012 study of a modified traditional inkblot paradigm actually demon-strated a high inter-rater reliability (0.88) among 16 examiners of 50 Rorschach records.[3] Inter-rater reliability can be determined by calcu-lating a Cohen's kappa rather than a Pearson's correlation coefficient, if our reliability data is categorical and dimensional.[4]

Test–retest reliability

Test–retest reliability is a measure of a test's reliability across time. A health-science example of a class of tests that have high test–retest reli-ability is IQ tests, which tend to be reliable across time because they test phenomena that tend to be constant across time. The Thurstone mental abilities test, for example, demonstrated test–retest reliability coefficients for five subscales between 0.77 and 0.82 over a test–retest interval of 21 years (1956 to 1977).[5]

Split-half reliability and Cronbach's alpha

Tests in and outside the health sciences vary enormously in their internal consistency and split-half reliability, and Cronbach's alpha can be used to reveal these levels. Split-half reliability is a measure of reliability between one half of the test and the other half. Cronbach's alpha was developed by Lee Cronbach in 1951[6] and is a measure of all possible split-half reliabilities. This reliability measure is commonly used in the health sciences, as well as in many other applications.

A new test measuring nursing competency in the operating theatre developed by researchers at the University of Melbourne provides an interesting example of the application of a Cronbach's alpha. It achieved a high Cronbach's alpha coefficient of item reliability.[7] A high between-item Cronbach's alpha of 0.94 was calculated for this performance-based scoring rubric.

Validity

What do you think makes a clinical test valid? As with reliability, the technical meaning of validity is exactly the same as the general meaning: a test, like an idea or a friend, is valid if it is *true*. And like a friend or an idea, a clinical test is true simply if it really means what it seems to mean. A test is valid, then, to the extent that it measures what it is *supposed* to measure, which is obviously important if a test is to be meaningful in the health sciences, including clinically meaningful.

There are different *measures* of validity, but there are not different *types* of validity. A test is either valid or it is not valid, in the same sense that a statement is either true or it is not true. What may appear to be different types of validity are actually different types of evidence of a test's validity and are commonly known as face validity, content validity, criterion validity and construct validity.

Face validity

This refers to the extent to which a test *appears* to measure what it is supposed to measure. This might seem like a superficial way of assessing the validity of a test, or anything else, but in practice if a test lacks face validity this can cause problems, such as reducing the motivation and level of cooperation of the person taking the test. Face validity could be seen as *apparent* as opposed to *actual* content validity.

A general health-science example of a test that lacks face validity is the so-called 'dolphin stress test' (DST), a jest test that is freely available on the internet. In this 'test', you are shown a photo that purports to be of two dolphins leaping out of the sea, but in fact the photo is of a dolphin and a cow. You are instructed that the more stressed you are, the less alike the two dolphins look!

A real health-science example of a test that achieved a far higher face validity than the DST is the self-medication assessment tool (SMAT). The test was for application to a geriatric population who may have cognitive deficits affecting their ability to self-manage their medication, and was trialled by a group of pharmacists. The results of the study showed that the pharmacists considered the test to have a sufficiently high face validity to justify using it.[8]

Content validity

Content validity refers to the relevance of a test to the construct that it purports to measure. An extreme example of a test that has high content validity is one that can successfully distinguish 'chalk' from 'cheese' (Fig 13.2). To assess a test's content validity, we need to assess the evidence that the test items are representative of the content domain (construct) being tested. Many health sciences commonly use constructs (such as stress) rather than the more tangible and directly measurable phenomena that are the domain of the physical sciences (such as physical objects).

The previously mentioned dolphin stress test (DST) lacks content validity because it lacks evidence that any of its items are related to the content of the construct — stress — that it purports to measure.

A real health-science example of a test that has demonstrated *high* content validity is the Aboriginal culture engagement survey. This test was developed as an important step in establishing an association between

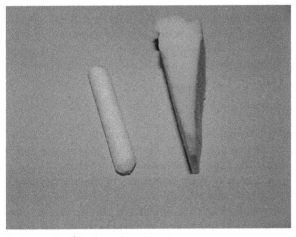

Fig 13.2   **The 'chalk or cheese' test**

culture and health benefits for a group of people who have particularly high health needs.[9]

Criterion validity

Criterion validity refers to a test's validity in terms of how its results compare with results on another relevant measure (criterion) of the construct it purports to measure. Criterion validity can be measured by calculating correlation coefficients of the associations between a test's measures and the criterion test's measures.

Predictive validity is a type of criterion validity that typically uses a future measure of performance, such as school or professional achievement or future medical outcome, as a measure. A diagnostic screen might be validated against an eventual medical outcome, for example.

Concurrent validity is a type of criterion validity that typically uses a current measure of performance, such as performance on a similar widely accepted test, as a measure. For example, a newly developed medical screen, such as one for dementia, could be assessed against a concurrently administered widely accepted screen, such as the mini-mental status examination.[10]

Again the DST is an example of a test that lacks both predictive and concurrent validity. There is no evidence that scores on this test are associated with eventual stress-related performance ability or with results on widely accepted concurrent stress measures, such as the Spielberger state–trait anxiety inventory.[11]

A real health-science example of the usefulness of calculating criterion validity is provided by a study that investigated the interesting question, 'Can people fake emotional intelligence (EI)?'.[12] This would appear to be an easier thing to fake than intellectual intelligence and could have interesting repercussions. The authors of this study used structural equation modelling to investigate the extent to which self-report measures of EI are susceptible to socially desirable responding. The results revealed that the criterion validity of EI for predicting life satisfaction, psychological distress and rational coping was lower in situations where faking was maximised — that is, when there was a high social desirability of achieving high scores on EI.

Construct validity

This refers to how valid a test is in terms of the validity of the construct that the test purports to be testing. What quantitative and qualitative evidence is there that the test constructor's underlying theory or model is valid? This evidence can again be assessed by examining correlation coefficients, in this case between scores on the test of interest and scores on tests that are supposed to have similar and also dissimilar constructs.

Convergent validity is a type of construct validity that will be high if, for example, scores on one stress test correlate strongly and positively with scores on other stress tests, which would support the validity of the stress construct.

Discriminant validity is a type of construct validity that will be high if scores on the items of a test do not correlate with scores on tests of dissimilar constructs, or correlate strongly and negatively with scores on tests of opposing constructs — for example, if scores on a stress test correlate negatively with scores on a relaxation test.

The DST is an example of a test that relates to a construct with high construct validity. Although we have previously maligned this test because it lacks many other forms of validity, it is actually high in construct validity in that it tests a construct for which there is a great deal of research evidence — stress.

An example of a construct that perhaps has less construct validity than it is generally thought to have is intelligence. This construct is believed, at least by some, including the IQ testing pioneer Charles Spearman, to be so diverse as to be meaningless.[13]

Test item construction

A test's overall reliability and validity depends on the reliability and validity of its individual items. Item analysis statistics are important for the development, improvement and evaluation of tests in the health sciences, and are the basis for improving tests through the selection, substitution and revision of their items. Information based on the item analysis of a test can be used to help shorten it, while at the same time improving its reliability and validity by eliminating items that do not perform well (for example, those having low reliability or validity). Some criteria for identifying test items that need purging are the following:

1. **Item difficulty.** This indicates the percentage of testees who answer an item correctly. Items should not be so hard that most testees get them wrong, or so easy that most testees get them right. The best wheat–chaff separating items are those of moderate difficulty.

2. **Item reliability.** This indicates the individual items that best measure what the entire scale measures and that also produce an appropriately wide range of scores. We can calculate item reliability by multiplying an item-total correlation by that item's standard deviation.

3. **Item validity.** This indicates the relationship of individual test items with a particular criterion, such as a gold standard of clinical diagnosis. We can calculate an item's validity by multiplying its correlation with a criterion variable and its standard deviation.

4. **Item discrimination.** A good test item is one that discriminates well between high and low test scorers.

Norms

Normative data is the performance data from a group of people who have previously taken a test or tests. This data can be used comparatively to provide meaning to the performance of people who are currently taking the same test or tests. Norms relate to standardisation (see Chapter 2). It does not mean much to say that a person scored 10 or 20 or even 20,000 on a test, but it does mean something to say that a person scored higher or lower than a relevant comparison group — for example, other people in the entire population, or other people in relevant strata of the entire population, such as people of a similar age, socioeconomic status or level of health to that of the person who is being tested.

Norms are also related to sampling principles (see Chapter 5), in that in order to properly compare a person's test score with a population summary score, the normative group must properly represent the population to which the individual belongs. We typically compare a person's test score with normative population scores by determining the number of standard deviation units separating their score from the normative mean.

Like many things, norms are often imperfect, so we need to be prudent in our interpretation of test scores against normative scores. We need to ask whether there is an appropriate norm to which we can compare our test results, and we also need to assess the quality of the normative data. How large was the normative sample? Is it relevant to the particular person or people whose results interest us? We also should remember that, like most things, norms change over time. For example, since formal intelligence testing began in the early 1900s, intelligence test scores have been increasing (known as the Flynn effect).[14] This may or may not mean that we are getting more intelligent, or that we are getting better at taking intelligence tests, but the implication for evaluating the appropriateness of normative groups for intelligence tests is that if we do not use recently tested normative groups we may overestimate people's intelligence, as is illustrated by the following example.

An example of changing norms

An interesting example of the effects of changes in norm groups is provided by the Rey auditory verbal learning test (RAVLT), which was developed in France in 1964 and which is still widely used for neuropsychological evaluation, including assessing brain damage. If we assess a person's performance against their professional occupation group norm by using the original 1964 French norms, and then assess them again using the 1990 Australian norms,[15] the same score on each assessment could be interpreted as signifying brain damage according to the original norms but normal according to the more recent norms. This could mean that French people are more intelligent than Australians, or that people internationally are less intelligent than they used to be, but it is more likely that some systematic distortions are involved here, and we always need to consider the possibility of this when interpreting scores against their norms. The original version of the RAVLT was translated from French into English, and this may well have affected the difficulty level of its items in the English translation. This illustrates an important principle of both statistical and life literacy — it is vital to look deeper than at appearances.

Conclusion

In this chapter you have been introduced to some important general test-related statistics that are very useful in the health sciences, as well as in many other applications. In the next and final chapter we will examine some statistics packages in action. This will be your chance to enter the statistical learner driver's seat, as you are guided through some widely used and useful computer statistics packages.

Quick reference summary

- In order to determine just how good a new or existing clinical test is, we need to know about some of its important characteristics, such as its reliability, validity and norms.

- The technical meaning of reliability is actually exactly the same as the everyday meaning, and this can usefully be defined as constancy or consistency.

- The technical meaning of validity is actually exactly the same as the everyday meaning: a test, like an idea or a friend, is valid if it is *true*.

- Normative data is the performance data from a group of people who have previously taken a test or tests. This data can be used to provide meaning for the scores of people who are currently taking the test or tests.

References

1. Spearman CC. Correlation calculated from faulty data. *British Journal of Psychology*. 1910;3:271-295.

2. Brown W. Some experimental results in the correlation of mental abilities. *British Journal of Psychology*. 1910;3:296-322.

3. Viglione DJ, Blume-Marcovici AC, Miller HL, et al. An inter-rater reliability study for the Rorschach performance assessment system. *Journal Personality Assessment*. 2012. [Epub ahead of print.]

4. Streiner DL, Norman GR. *PDQ Epidemiology*. 3rd ed. Shelton, CT: People's Medical Publishing House; 2009.

5. Hertzog C, Schaie KW. Stability and change in adult intelligence: 2. Simultaneous analysis of longitudinal means and covariance structures. *Psychological Aging*. 1988;3(2)[Jun]:130-132.

6. Cronbach LJ. Coefficient alpha and the internal structure of tests. *Psychometrika*. 1951;16(3):297-334.

7. Nicholson P, Griffin P, Gillis S, et al. Measuring nursing competencies in the operating theatre: instrument development and psychometric analysis using Item Response Theory. *Nursing Education Today*. 2012. [Epub ahead of print.]

8. Irvine-Meek J, Gould ON, Wheaton H, et al. Acceptability and face validity of a geriatric self-medication assessment tool. *Canadian Journal of Hospital Pharmacy*. 2010;63(3) [May]:225-232.

9. Berry SL, Crowe TP, Deane FP. Preliminary development and content validity of a measure of Australian Aboriginal cultural engagement. *Ethnic Health*. 2012. [Epub ahead of print.]

10. Folstein M, Folstein S, McHugh P. 'Mini mental state': a practical method for grading the cognitive state of patients for the clinician. *Journal of Psychiatric Research*. 1975;13:189-198.

11. Spielberger CD, Gorsuch RL, Lushene RE. *Manual for the State–Trait Anxiety Inventory*. Palo Alto, Calif: Consulting Psychologists Press; 1970.

12. Choi S, Kluemper DH, Sauley KS. What if we fake emotional intelligence? A test of criterion validity attenuation. *Journal of Personality Assessment*. 2011;93(3)[May]:270-277.

13. Spearman C. Some issues in the theory of 'g' (including the Law of Diminishing Returns). *Nature*. 1925;116(2916):436-439.

14. Nisbett RE, Aronson J, Blair C, et al. Intelligence: new findings and theoretical developments. *American Psychology*. 2012;67(2)[Feb-Mar]:130-159. [Epub 2 Jan 2012].

15. Geffen G, Moar KJ, O'Hanlon AP, et al. Performance measures of 16- to 86-year-old males and females on the Auditory Verbal Learning Test. *The Clinical Neuropsychologist*. 1990;4:45-63.

Further reading

Cronbach LJ, Shavelson RJ. My current thoughts on coefficient alpha and successor procedures. *Educational and Psychological Measurement*. 2004;64(3)[Jun 1]:391-418.

CHAPTER 14

STATISTICS AND THE COMPUTER
Dean McKenzie

The journey is the thing.
HOMER

OBJECTIVES

After carefully reading this chapter you will have an understanding of:

- the importance of computers in the statistical analysis of data, as well as some of the exciting developments currently going on in the world of statistical computing

- four of the main general statistical packages used in the health sciences

- the basic steps to be taken before embarking on statistical journeys with a computer

- the comparative ease of using a computer package rather than a pen and paper (or quill and parchment) to calculate statistics.

Introduction

Computers have long been a boon to statisticians. Even back when they (the computers, not the statisticians) occupied whole rooms and weighed several tonnes (Fig 14.1), statistical software was developed to perform statistical calculations.[1]

Performing statistical tests by hand can genuinely aid understanding of the underlying principles of statistics, but can also be tedious, or even practically impossible in the case of larger data sets or more complex procedures, such as multiple linear regression and logistic regression (see Chapter 10). Nowadays, there is a computer on almost every desk, making it theoretically possible for almost everyone to perform statistical analyses easily (something of a mixed blessing). Nevertheless, computers and computational techniques allow modern health scientists to ask and find answers to questions that previously would have been impossible to answer. As computer-assisted statistical capacity becomes ever more available, it allows new insights into the masses of data that are being collected all around us — in laboratories, hospitals, residences, shopping malls and even on the internet.

Bootstrapping

The development of ever faster computers has led to the development of what are often called computer-intensive statistical methods.[2] One such

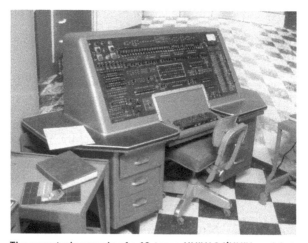

Fig 14.1 The operator's console of a 13-tonne UNIVAC I (UNIVersal Automatic Computer I) mainframe computer, first produced in 1951. Unlike most human pollsters, a UNIVAC I computer correctly predicted that Dwight D Eisenhower (1890-1969) would win the 1952 US presidential election by a landslide, defeating Adlai Ewing Stevenson II (1900-65).[1]

method is the 'bootstrap', named and developed in the 1970s by Bradley Efron.[3] The bootstrap extends earlier work by researchers such as Julian Lincoln Simon (1932–98)[4] and John Wilder Tukey (1915–2000),[5] the latter of whom invented the term 'software' (as in computer software), among many other things.[6] Earlier work, in the related area of permutation tests defined below, was performed by the Australian researcher Edwin James George Pitman (1897–1993),[7] as well as by Sir Ronald Aylmer Fisher (1890–1962).[8]

Bootstrapping resembles repeating an experiment many times in order to get an idea of the variability in the results. Rather than actually rerunning the experiment many times, which would require a great deal of time and money, the bootstrapping technique generates many thousands of subsamples that are randomly selected, or 'resampled', by computer from the original sample or data set. For example, if the original sample contained three observations (which of course would be rare in reality), the first bootstrap subsample may contain the first observation, two copies of the second observation and none at all of the third observation; the second bootstrap subsample may consist of three copies of the second observation, and so on. The particular result of interest (a median or a kappa coefficient, for example) is recorded for each subsample and tallied. With a little more processing by the computer, a confidence interval can be obtained, based upon the empirical distribution of the actual subsamples, rather than on a theoretical normal distribution.

The bootstrap is used in many health-science applications, such as for testing whether a type of anxiety disorder observed in adolescents ought to constitute a new diagnostic category,[9] or identifying successful preoperative risk factors for 30-day mortality following cardiac surgery in Australian patients.[10] The bootstrap has been used in various applications in this author's own research, including comparing the performance of depression screening tests in Australian hospital patients (which also involved the use of permutation tests), and predicting future depression in Australian and American adolescents.[11,12] Some of the methodological aspects of the research have recently been extended by other workers in the field to allow comparison of three or more screening tests, for example.[13]

Permutation tests

Another computer-intensive resampling technique is known as 'permutation tests' (also called randomisation tests), which involve permuting or reordering scores. For example, imagine that three people, Alpha, Bravo and Charlie, have been randomly assigned to a particular experimental condition, while three other people, Delta, Echo and Foxtrot, have been randomly assigned to a placebo condition (the original permutation tests being built around the idea of random assignment to experimental and control conditions). At the end of our study, the number of people who did and did not become ill (for example) are tallied and the counts compared. But what difference in counts would be obtained if we relabelled the scores, so that Alpha, Bravo and Charlie were in the placebo group and Delta, Echo and Foxtrot were in the experimental group?

In permutation tests we work out the difference or other statistic of interest for each possible rearrangement of scores to groups or condtions, and how often such results exceed or equal the result that we actually obtained. The number of possible arrangements can soon become astronomical. Although there are only 20 ways of assigning 6 people to 2 groups of 3 each, there are 137,846,528,820 ways of assigning 40 people to 2 groups of 20 each, using the combination rule for calculating the number of ways that r 'things' (such as 3 people) can be selected from n 'things' (such as 6 people)![14] When every possible rearrangement or permutation is calculated, generally using sophisticated computer algorithms, permutation tests are known as 'exact permutation tests', or sometimes just 'exact tests'.

The statistical test for comparing counts of categorical data (originally intended only for binary data; see Chapter 7) — generally known as Fisher's exact test — is a comparatively well-known example of an exact test. When there are simply too many permutations for even the fastest computers to compute, we might simply randomly choose 10,000 or so of the billions, trillions or squillions of the possible permutations. Such tests are known as Monte Carlo permutation tests.[2,15] In the case of categorical data, exact and Monte Carlo permutation tests are often used when an assumption of the chi-square test, that the expected counts for each cell of the table are sufficiently large (see Chapter 7), does not hold. Permutation tests have been employed in a variety of health-science applications,[16] including studies of Australian hospital patients[17] and Australian war veterans.[18,19] The latter applications involved exact permutation versions[20] of logistic regression (see Chapter 10 for discussion of the general form of logistic regression).

Although permutation tests, and the arguably even more flexible bootstrap technique,[3] are not intended as answers to all our statistical (or other) problems, and although they are a little more complex than they may first appear, the above outline may, hopefully, have whetted your appetite for more of what is being undertaken in the world of statistical computing. But first you need to gain some experience using statistical packages applied to some statistical 'bread and butter', or building-blocks, such as the t-test and the Pearson product-moment correlation. Statistical packages can be defined as software that can readily perform many different statistical tests, and they make the tasks of researchers much easier, when it comes to analysing data at least!

Statistical packages

Many wonderful statistical packages are available, but for reasons of space and simplicity an overview of four general statistical packages commonly employed in the Health Sciences — IBM® SPSS®, SAS®, Stata® and R — is presented here. All four packages are long established (the large computer or 'mainframe' versions of IBM® SPSS® and SAS® were originally developed in the 1960s) and yet still remain leading-edge. If you are going to analyse data by computer, you will need to gain an understanding of at least one statistical package.

IBM® SPSS®

The letters SPSS originally stood for **S**tatistical **P**ackage for the **S**ocial **S**ciences. SPSS was bought by IBM in 2009 and is now known as IBM® SPSS® (it was also briefly known as Predictive Analytics Software [PASW]). IBM® SPSS® has always been very well regarded for its ease of use, and recent versions of this package provide many more statistical and programming features than earlier versions. For example, mixed or multilevel models for hierarchical structures (such as of patients within wards, within hospitals) or repeated measurements across time[21,22] mentioned in Chapter 8 are available in recent versions of IBM® SPSS®.

At the time of writing, however, IBM® SPSS® is not able to perform some contemporary statistical techniques, such as robust regression,[23] which is intended for use on data containing extreme scores or outliers. In principle, robust regression resembles Spearman's rank–order correlation (outlined in Chapter 9), although the former can be used with more than one predictor and generally does not require the data to be ranked.[23] Furthermore, some of the IBM® SPSS® procedures currently lack the ability to directly compute confidence intervals. For example, confidence intervals for Pearson product-moment correlations using the Fisher's z transformation (see Chapter 9) can easily be calculated by R or Stata® or SAS®, but not directly by IBM® SPSS®. The latter package would require a small amount of programming, or the use of the add-on bootstrap module. Such a module might, depending on your IBM® SPSS® installation, be an extra-cost option.

Programming the Fisher's z confidence interval method in IBM® SPSS® is reasonably straightforward, providing that one knows how to use the IBM® SPSS® command language syntax. Even within R, more sophisticated procedures such as the bootstrap, briefly outlined at the outset of this chapter, may be needed to obtain confidence intervals for other correlation coefficients such as Spearman's correlation.[24]

IBM® SPSS® is arguably the easiest to learn of the statistical packages outlined in this chapter, in terms of statistical analysis and data transformations, but if you choose it as your main statistical package, you may need to use another package — such as SAS®, Stata® or R — for more specialised analyses or for data programming. This is rather like using a second language such as French when the right word is not available in English ('gourmand', for example). As an alternative to using two different statistical packages, IBM® SPSS® now allows statistical procedures such as robust regression to be called up from the freely available R statistical package (discussed below), using various steps.[25]

Interested (and hopefully also disinterested) readers can find more details on IBM® SPSS® on its official website at <http://www-01.ibm.com/software/analytics/spss/> and in the books listed in Further Reading at the end of this chapter. Specially priced versions of IBM® SPSS® and other statistical software (but not SAS® or Stata®) — intended for eligible students and academics — are available at <http://www.onthehub.com/>. A general website that contains much useful information on IBM® SPSS® can be found at <http://www.ats.ucla.edu/stat/spss/>.

SAS®

The letters SAS® originally stood for **S**tatistical **A**nalysis **S**ystem. SAS® is often regarded as the world's most widely used statistical package[26] and is frequently employed in government and industry (particularly the pharmaceutical industry), as well as in the health sciences.

SAS® and IBM® SPSS® are often thought to be similar to each other.[27] Although SAS® is arguably more difficult to use than is IBM® SPSS®, it is also arguably more powerful. For example, SAS® has more regression routines than IBM® SPSS®, including robust regression. The SAS® programming command language for creating and recoding variables is also more powerful than that of IBM® SPSS®.[27] As with IBM® SPSS®, if SAS® cannot do something for you, you can use another statistical package for a specific analysis, or call up statistical routines from R, within SAS®.[25]

Interested readers can find more details about SAS® on its official website <http://www.sas.com/> and in the books listed in Further Reading at the end of this chapter. A general website that contains lots of useful information on SAS® is <http://www.ats.ucla.edu/stat/sas/>.

Stata®

New versions of statistical packages are usually released every year or two. In between these releases, users throughout the world are developing new statistical procedures, often for the packages that they themselves use. Such user-written procedures can be found, installed and performed for all four of the statistical packages outlined here, but is much easier to do this in Stata® and R than it is in IBM® SPSS® and SAS®. For example, it is possible to search the internet for user-written Stata® statistical procedures from within Stata® itself, using the Stata® 'findit' command, and then install them. Similar operations are more indirect in IBM® SPSS® and SAS®. Furthermore, most new statistical books and papers include user-written statistical procedures for Stata® and/or R.[28]

Stata® (along with SAS® and R) can readily do many things, particularly in regard to regression analysis, that IBM® SPSS® cannot do easily, if at all. On the other hand, Stata® is far more particular than IBM® SPSS® and SAS® about typing commands correctly. For example, if Stata® asks for something to be typed in lower case, then it really *must* be typed in lower case, and the same applies to R.

While arguably more flexible than IBM® SPSS® or SAS® when it comes to adding new procedures, Stata® is also a commercial package, and so a lot of support is available, including an official dial-up helpline to ask questions (IBM® SPSS® and SAS® also have official helplines). There is also an independent Statalist facility, where you can electronically post a question and someone, somewhere, will (generally) answer it for you.

If Stata® really cannot do something for you, you may be able to do it using another statistical package. Although Stata® (unlike IBM® SPSS® and SAS®) does not yet have inbuilt facilities for directly using R routines, user-written Stata® procedures for calling up R are available.[28]

Interested readers can find more details about Stata® at the official US website at <http://www.stata.com/> or the Australian distributor's website at <http://www.survey-design.com.au/>, as well as in the books listed in 'Further reading' at the end of this chapter. A general website that contains a lot of useful information on Stata® can be found at <http://www.ats.ucla.edu/stat/stata/>. Statalist is hosted at the Harvard University School of Public Health, at <http://www.stata.com/statalist/>.

R

R is a 'workalike' variation of a statistical package/programming language called S, commercially available as S-PLUS® (now known as TIBCO Spotfire S+® Advanced Stats; see <http://spotfire.tibco.com/~/media/content-center/datasheets/advanced-stats.ashx> and <http://www.solutionmetrics.com.au/products/splus/default.html>). R was developed in New Zealand by **R**obert Gentleman and **R**oss Ihaka (hence the name R) and is free as in free speech, as well as being free as in free lemonade. Third-party commercial versions of R exist,[25] but any costs are associated with the provided support, or a friendlier user interface than the more basic one generally provided with R. The commercial S-PLUS® package includes a sophisticated user interface.

The 'source code' to R, or the actual programming routines in which it is written, must always be allowed to be distributed, extended and viewed, which is what is generally meant by the term 'open source' when describing software such as R. R is growing as quickly as the proverbial Topsy, with thousands of statistical routines (known perhaps confusingly as 'packages' within R) available at <http://cran.r-project.org/web/packages/>.

Such routines can easily be downloaded and installed directly from within R itself.

R is often regarded as a statistical common language, or *lingua franca*.[25] If someone develops a snazzy new statistical procedure, for example, he or she might implement it in R, so that it can be available to anyone with a computer, an internet connection and a practical interest in using that particular procedure (perhaps in order to help answer a particular research question). If the new procedure were to be written for IBM® SPSS®, SAS® or Stata®, however, only people with access to those commercial packages could use it. This is a wonderful feature of R, but it also brings up questions of the accuracy and validity of its statistical procedures. Favourable evidence of the validity of R has been presented,[25] but an evaluative eye (at least) should be kept on the use of R procedures, particularly in regard to the selection of statistical options.[29] Where possible, it is wise to employ R routines that are described in highly regarded books and journals, and to consult with statisticians who are familiar with different statistical techniques and their implementations.

IBM® SPSS®, SAS® and Stata® offer point-and-click graphic user interfaces as well as the option of keying in commands. R, however, requires commands to be keyed in, but free (as in speech, beer and lemonade) graphic interfaces are available separately for R, such as Rcmdr (R Commander) and Rattle (R Analytic Tool to Learn Easily).

Interested readers can find more details on R on its official website <http://cran.r-project.org/> and in the books listed in Further Reading at the end of this chapter. R is increasingly being employed in health-science applications,[30] with one study applying both R and Stata® to examine the relationship between air pollution levels and out-of-hospital heart attacks in Melbourne.[31] A general website with much useful information about R can be found at <http://www.ats.ucla.edu/stat/R/>. As R can be a little daunting for the new (and occasionally old) user, a helpful introductory website can be found at <http://www.statmethods.net/>. Rcmdr is available at <http://socserv.mcmaster.ca/jfox/Misc/Rcmdr/>. Rattle is available at <http://www.rattle.togaware.com>.

Which statistical package(s) should I learn and use?

Many books are entirely devoted to just one statistical package, and so one chapter cannot hope to do justice to four statistical packages, let alone to other packages or specialist statistical computer programs (many of which are listed at <http://www.stata.com/links/stat_software.html>.

Overall, of the four statistical packages discussed above, IBM® SPSS® is arguably the easiest to learn and use. SAS®, Stata® and especially R are arguably more powerful but also more difficult to learn than IBM® SPSS®.

This is especially true when R is employed for more advanced analyses or data programming. Your own personal choice of package(s) to learn should be based upon factors such as suitability for your present and future projects, ease of use, availability, cost and what your colleagues are using.

Some caveats for computer analysis

Before actually calculating some statistical tests using a computer, bear the following suggestions in mind.

There is always one more bug!

Data that are supposedly error-free will usually still have errors. Always perform checks for unlikely values — not only for single variables, but also for combinations of variables (such as looking for pregnant males).

Be patient!

Real data are rarely found in a form suitable for statistical analysis, and a lot of analysis time is actually spent getting data ready for statistical analysis. One might, for example, need to create a variable representing whether or not a particular disease or disorder is present, based upon the presence or absence of many symptoms. This is generally accomplished using data transformation commands, available in all the packages outlined above. Once errors have been identified and hopefully fixed, and any recoding done or variables created, statistical analysis (like many things) generally takes much longer than expected. Something to avoid, wherever possible, is just 'running the results through the computer to see if they are significant'. This is a similar process to going on statistical fishing expeditions, as mentioned in previous chapters, instead of becoming thoroughly acquainted with the data. Statistical significance should not be an end in itself.[32] Thorough understanding of our data, in a valid and replicable fashion, should always be our quest!

Leave a record for posterity!

As well as keeping an analytic diary or logbook, it really *is* necessary to keep electronic records of all the data transformation and statistical commands that you have used, so that someone else, or you yourself a week or a year later, can easily replicate your analyses. Even though it has been sagely asked (by an unknown graffiti artist) 'What has posterity done for me?', we can do a great deal for posterity. Merely selecting choices from a computer menu may make it hard to record what specific analytical steps were taken, and may reduce our analytical flexibility compared with what could be achieved using more direct commands.[33,34] Just think of the 'contemporary' telephone inquiry systems that allow us to specify what we actually want, rather than having to go through all those menus.

Never fly solo!

Acquiring and checking data generally takes a great deal of time and financial resources, so data are always worth analysing properly. This generally means working under the guidance of experienced statisticians, as even seemingly simple analyses can have hidden traps. It is safest to meet with a statistician before the study or project is conducted, as well as before you begin analysing data, and then regularly thereafter. Please be aware, however, that statisticians are generally busy on lots of other projects and so are therefore seldom free in the sense of 'available', so you will need to allow plenty of time. Also, in these days of academic funding uncertainty, university statistical consulting services are usually not free (as in lemonade), although some academic institutions may set aside a number of hours for statistical support for postgraduate research students.

Conclusion

This chapter has provided you with a taste of what can be accomplished using computers to perform statistical analysis. At this stage, though, the process may be a little like setting out to learn a few 'helpful' travel phrases, such as 'please tell me what time the hovercraft leaves?', without knowing the follow-up questions, such as 'and could I have a seat by the window please?' In a similar fashion to gaining skill in human languages, gaining skill in computer statistical packages requires much learning, patience and, above all, much practice. Details of classroom or web-based courses may be available from your local university, or one nearby, or from a national research body such as <http://www.acspri.org.au/>, as well as from the websites of IBM® SPSS®, SAS® and Stata® provided above. Web-based courses on R, as well as the above packages, are also available from commercial websites such as <http://www.statistics.com>.

Some great guides to the statistical packages outlined here are listed in Further Reading. It is also strongly suggested that you buy, or borrow, another excellent book that has been the mainstay of applied statisticians and health-science researchers for almost 30 years, and is currently in its sixth edition. This book, which is brimful of practical suggestions and advice for analysing data by computer, is *Using Multivariate Statistics* by Barbara Tabachnick and Linda Fidell.[22]

Quick reference summary

- Computers can relieve the tedium involved in applying simple techniques to both simple and large data sets. They also facilitate the use of complex procedures such as multiple linear regression and logistic regression, as well as computer-intensive procedures such as permutation tests and the bootstrap.

- Four of the most commonly employed general statistical packages — the commercial software IBM® SPSS®, SAS®, Stata® and the open-source, freely available R — are broadly examined in this chapter.

- IBM® SPSS® may not be as powerful or comprehensive as the other packages outlined in this chapter, particularly in the case of techniques such as robust regression, but it is arguably easier to use than the other packages.

- Be *patient* in analysing data, making sure that data are free from errors, allowing time to check for this and to recode or create variables needed in the actual analyses. Meet regularly with statistical experts and do not simply rush to find 'significant' results!

- Choose at least one statistical package to work with, buy or borrow statistical books and take statistical courses as required.

- Get some hands-on experience, preferably with your own data (and your own hands), or at least with data that you found on the web or in a book and that looks interesting.

References

1. Hally M. *Electronic Brains: Stories from the Dawn of the Computer Age*. London: Granta; 2005.

2. Manly BFJ. *Randomization, Bootstrap and Monte Carlo Methods in Biology*. 3rd ed. Boca Raton, FL: Chapman & Hall/CRC; 2006.

3. Efron B, Tibshirani RJ. *An Introduction to the Bootstrap*. New York: Chapman and Hall; 1993.

4. Simon JL. *Basic Research Methods in Social Science*. New York: Random House; 1969.

5. Tukey JW. Bias and confidence in not quite large samples (abstract). *Annals of Mathematical Statistics*. 1958;29:64.

6. Wainer H. *Graphic Display: a Trout in the Milk and Other Visual Adventures*. Princeton, NJ: Princeton University Press; 2005.

7. Pitman EJG. Significance tests which may be applied to samples from any populations. *Journal of The Royal Statistical Society*. 1937;4(supplement):119-130.

8. Fisher RA. *The Design of Experiments*. Edinburgh: Oliver & Boyd; 1935.

9. Schmidt NB, Kotov R, Bernstein A, et al. Mixed anxiety depression: taxometric exploration of the validity of a diagnostic category in youth. *Journal of Affective Disorders*. 2007;98:83-89.

10. Billah B, Reid CM, Shardey GC, et al. A preoperative risk prediction model for 30-day mortality following cardiac surgery in an Australian cohort. *European Journal of Cardiothoracic Surgery*. 2010;37:1086-1092.

11. McKenzie DP, Mackinnon AJ, Peladeau N, et al. Comparing correlated kappas by resampling: is one level of agreement significantly different from another? *Journal of Psychiatric Research*. 1996;30:483-492.

12. McKenzie DP, Toumbourou JW, Forbes AB, et al. Predicting future depression in adolescents using the Short Mood and Feelings Questionnaire: a two-nation study. *Journal of Affective Disorders*. 2011;134:151-159.

13. Vanbelle S, Albert A. A bootstrap method for comparing correlated kappa coefficients. *Journal of Statistical Computation and Simulation*. 2008;78:1009-1015.

14. Bluman AG. *Probability Demystified*. 2nd ed. New York: McGraw-Hill; 2012.

15. Mehta CR. The exact analysis of contingency tables in medical research. *Statistical Methods in Medical Research*. 1994;3:135-156.

16. Morita A, Nakayama T, Soma M. Association study between C-reactive protein genes and ischemic stroke in Japanese subjects. *American Journal of Hypertension*. 2006;19:593-600.

17. Clarke DM, Smith GC, Dowe DL, et al. An empirically derived taxonomy of common distress syndrome in the medically ill. *Journal of Psychosomatic Research*. 2003;54:323-330.

18. Ikin JF, Sim MR, Creamer MC, et al. War-related psychological stressors and risk of psychological disorders in Australian veterans of the 1991 Gulf War. *British Journal of Psychiatry*. 2004;185:116-126.

19. McKenzie DP, Ikin JF, McFarlane AC, et al. Psychological health of Australian veterans of the 1991 Gulf War: an assessment using the SF-12, GHQ-12 and PCL-S. *Psychological Medicine*. 2004;34:1419-1430.

20. Mehta CR, Patel NR. Exact logistic regression: theory and examples. *Statistics in Medicine*. 1995;14:2143-2160.

21. Field A. *Discovering Statistics Using SPSS*. 3rd ed. Thousand Oaks, CA: Sage; 2009.

22. Tabachnick BG, Fidell LS. *Using Multivariate Statistics*. 6th ed. Upper Saddle River, NJ: Pearson; 2013.

23. Andersen R. *Modern Methods for Robust Regression*. Thousand Oaks, CA: Sage; 2008.

24. Wright DB, London K. *Modern Regression Techniques Using R: a Practical Guide for Students and Researchers*. Thousand Oaks, CA: Sage; 2009.

25. Muenchen RA. *R for SAS and SPSS users*. 2nd ed. New York: Springer; 2011.

26. Der G, Everitt BS. *A Handbook of Statistical Analyses Using SAS*. 3rd ed. Boca Raton, FL: Chapman and Hall/CRC; 2009.

27. Delwiche LD, Slaughter SJ. *The Little SAS book: a Primer*. 4th ed. Cary, NC: SAS Institute; 2008.

28. Muenchen RA, Hilbe JM. *R for Stata Users*. New York: Springer; 2010.

29. Austin PC. R and S-PLUS produced different classification trees for predicting patient mortality. *Journal of Clinical Epidemiology*. 2008;61:1222-1226.

30. Watson R, van der Ark LA, Lin LC, et al. Item response theory: how Mokken scaling can be used in clinical practice. *Journal of Clinical Nursing*. 2012;21:2736:2746.

31. Dennekamp M, Akram M, Abramson MJ, et al. Outdoor air pollution as a trigger for out-of-hospital cardiac arrests. *Epidemiology*. 2010;21:494-500.

32. Cumming G. *Understanding the New Statistics: Effect Sizes, Confidence Intervals, and Meta-analysis*. New York: Routledge; 2012.

33. Collier J. *Using SPSS Syntax: a Beginner's Guide*. Thousand Oaks, CA: Sage; 2010.

34. Gordon RA. *Applied Statistics for the Social and Health Sciences*. New York: Routledge; 2012.

Further reading

IBM® SPSS®

Field A. *Discovering Statistics Using SPSS*. 3rd ed. Thousand Oaks, CA: Sage; 2009.

Pallant J. *SPSS Survival Manual: a Step by Step Guide to Data Analysis Using SPSS Windows (Version 18)*. 4th ed. Sydney: Allen & Unwin; 2011.

SAS®

Delwiche LD, Slaughter SJ. *The Little SAS Book: a Primer.* 4th ed. Cary, NC: SAS Institute; 2008.

Field A, Miles J. *Discovering Statistics Using SAS.* Thousand Oaks, CA: Sage; 2010.

Stata®

Longest KC. *Using Stata for Quantitative Analysis.* Thousand Oaks, CA: Sage; 2012.

Pevalin DJ. *The Stata Survival Manual.* Maidenhead: Open University Press; 2009.

R

Field A, Miles J, Field Z. *Discovering Statistics Using R.* Thousand Oaks, CA: Sage; 2012.

Verzani J. *Using R for Introductory Statistics.* Boca Raton, FL: Chapman & Hall/CRC; 2005.

General

Bentley PJ. *Digitized: the Science of Computers and How It Shapes Our World.* Oxford: Oxford University Press; 2012.

Shalizi C. The bootstrap. *American Scientist.* 2010;98:186-190.

Index

Page numbers followed by 'f' indicate figures, by 't' indicate tables, and by 'b' indicate boxes.

Lightning Source UK Ltd.
Milton Keynes UK
UKHW020718260722
406385UK00007B/422